THE EVERYTHING®

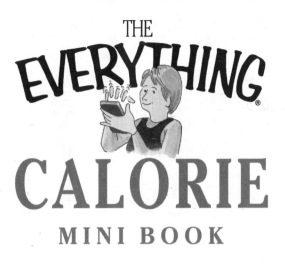

CALORIE

MINI BOOK

Barbara Ravage

Adams Media Corporation
Avon

An Everything® Series Book.
"Everything" is a registered trademark of Adams Media Corporation.

Published by Adams Media Corporation
57 Littlefield Street, Avon, MA 02322
www.adamsmedia.com

ISBN: 1-58062-607-6

Printed in Canada.

J I H G F E D C B A

Library of Congress Cataloging-in-Publication Data
available from the publisher.

This publication is designed to provide accurate and authoritative information with regard to the subject matter covered. It is sold with the under-
standing that the publisher is not engaged in rendering legal, accounting, or
other professional advice. If legal advice or other expert assistance is
required, the services of a competent professional person should be sought.
— From a *Declaration of Principles* jointly adopted by a Committee of the
American Bar Association and a Committee of Publishers and Associations

Many of the designations used by manufacturers and sellers to distinguish
their products are claimed as trademarks. Where those designations appear
in this book and Adams Media was aware of a trademark claim, the designations have been printed in initial capital letters.

Cover illustrations by Barry Littmann.
Interior illustrations by Barry Littmann.
Additional contributions by Susan Gaber.

Contents

Introduction

The Everything® Calorie Mini Book is designed as a compact reference, small enough to slip into your pocket or purse when you go to the supermarket or are eating away from home. It won't take up much space on your kitchen counter either, so you can refer to it when you are planning and preparing meals.

How to Use This Book

This book contains the calorie content of more than 3,000 foods and ingredients, organized in categories to make it easy to find what you're looking for. The main categories, arranged in alphabetical order, are:

1. Beverages, including alcoholic and soft drinks, as well as fruit and vegetable juices
2. Breads, crackers, and baked goods
3. Dairy and eggs, including milk and milk beverages
4. Diet and health foods
5. Extras, including dressings, gravies, sauces, condiments, flavorings, herbs, and spices
6. Fats and oils
7. Fish and seafood
8. Fruits
9. Cereals, grains, rice, pasta
10. Meats and poultry
11. Nuts and seeds
12. Snack foods

13. Soups, stews, casseroles, and other combination foods
14. Sweets and desserts, including common baking ingredients
15. Vegetables and dried beans

How to Find What You're Looking For

Within each category, foods are arranged by subcategories. For example, within "Meats and Poultry," you will find beef, pork, lamb, chicken, duck, turkey, and so on. And within those subcategories, you will find specific cuts of meat or poultry and methods of preparation.

In an effort to include as many foods as possible, branded items have been listed only when they are unique and cannot be covered by a general item. For example, cola is listed among soft drinks, but Dr. Pepper is listed by brand name. General listings are often averages of several brand-name items. For example, there are many different brands of yogurt and many give different names to their flavors: french vanilla or vanilla, mixed fruit or fruit medley, etc. Instead of listing them all, yogurts are distinguished by their fat content (whole milk, low fat, and no fat) and an average calorie count is used.

In all of these cases, if you are looking for an exact calorie count, look at the label on the product in question.

What You Won't Find

Because there are literally tens of thousands of different food products on supermarket shelves, no attempt has been made to list every item and every brand. In particular, special diet foods that are available in supermarkets as well as from weight-loss programs are too numerous to mention. Nonetheless, all of these items are labeled with their calorie content, allowing you to figure out how many calories you are consuming.

What Is a Calorie?

A calorie is a unit of energy. In the human body, this energy is used to build, repair, and maintain tissue (bone, muscle, and organs), and to fuel metabolism and activity. Energy that is not used is stored as fat. Approximately 3,500 calories add up to 1 pound of stored body fat.

In food, a calorie represents the amount of energy it provides when it is consumed, either for use or storage. There are three main nutrient types:

- *Carbohydrates,* which contain 4 calories per gram*
- *Proteins,* which contain 4 calories per gram*
- *Fats,* which contain 9 calories per gram*

A fourth type, *alcohol,* contains 7 calories per gram.* Alcoholic beverages are, therefore, relatively high in calories, and they are empty calories at that. Unlike fats, proteins, and carbohydrates, alcohol offers no nutritional benefit, nothing the body needs or can use for energy or to build cells.

Although this is useful information, the fact is few foods contain only a single nutrient type. Most are combinations, which is why you need a calorie counter such as this one.

*By weight, 28 grams equals 1 ounce.

How Many Calories Do You Need?

The number of calories an individual needs to maintain all body processes differs according to many variables. A person's activity level, gender, and current weight all influence how many calories are needed. The rate of metabolism also influences how calories are burned and stored in the body. Figuring out how much you need to keep your weight the same, or to lose or gain weight, involves some complicated calculations. Some general guidelines for maintaining weight (neither gaining nor losing) have been set, however. Use the table on the next page to see how many calories a person of your age, weight, and gender needs every day to stay the same weight.

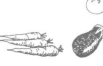

Recommended Calorie Intake
(by age, gender, and weight)

Age	Weight in pounds	Daily calorie intake
Infants		
to 6 months	13	650
6–12 months	20	850
Children		
1–3 years	29	1300
4–6 years	44	1800
7–10 years	52	2000
Teens, Female		
11–14 years	101	2200
15–18 years	120	2200
Teens, Male		
11–14 years	99	2500
15–18 years	145	3000

Recommended Calorie Intake
(continued)
(by age, gender, and weight)

Age	Weight in pounds	Daily calorie intake
Adults, Female		
19–24 years	128	2200
25–50 years	138	2200
51+ years	143	1900

Pregnant: add 300 calories/day for second and third trimester

Lactating: add 500 calories/day

Age	Weight in pounds	Daily calorie intake
Adults, Male		
19–24 years	160	2900
25–50 years	174	2900
51+ years	170	2300

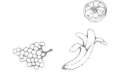

These are approximate figures only. If you want to figure out how many calories a person of your age, gender, height, weight, and activity levels needs, numerous weight-loss and nutrition sites on the Internet feature calculators for this purpose.

Losing weight, of course, is a more complicated matter. Theoretically, you can do this by reducing your calorie intake over a period of time at the rate of 3,500 calories per pound you wish to lose. It will be far more effective, realistic, and lasting to reduce calorie intake *and* increase your level of activity. You will not only lose weight—you will also look and feel better, and improve your overall health.

What Is a Serving?

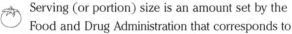

Serving (or portion) size is an amount set by the Food and Drug Administration that corresponds to

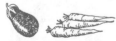

how much an average person would eat. All food labels are required by law to indicate the number of calories per serving, not per package or container. For people who are counting calories, *this is a very important point.*

A box of crackers contains more than one serving. If you imagine that the per-serving calorie count refers to the entire box, you will be in for a nasty surprise the next time you get on the scale. Likewise, many canned or bottled beverages contain more than a single serving. Moreover, muffins, bagels, and other baked goods vary in size and therefore calorie count. Finally, the values given in the alcoholic beverages section are approximate at best. Much depends on who's pouring and the proof (alcohol percentage) of what's being poured.

The best thing to do is to read labels, if possible, and do some number crunching on your own. The only way to be sure you are consuming

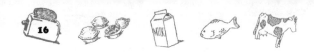

the number of calories you think you are is to pay attention to serving size.

You can measure servings in various ways. Sometimes it is a matter of counting pieces. Other times a measuring cup, spoon, or kitchen scale will give you the information you need. For packaged food, it may be a matter of dividing the contents into the number of servings it contains, and eating only one portion.

After a while, you will have a pretty good idea of what a serving of a particular food looks like. Still, it is a good idea to start out by measuring. Go back to measuring every once in a while to maintain accuracy. "Portion creep" is a major contributing factor to the failure of weight-loss plans and the problem of obesity in general.

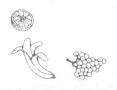

Read the Label!

According to the law, all packaged and prepared
foods must carry nutritional information, including
calorie content, on their labels. This includes foods
that come in boxes, cans, bottles, and numerous
other containers. Fresh fruits and vegetables,
unprocessed meats, and other "unpackaged" foods
are not included. Nonetheless, most of the foods
Americans buy and eat are covered by the label
law. Reading labels can give you a lot of useful
information, if you know how to look for it.

- Serving size is perhaps the most important
  piece of information you will find on a label.
  Except for single-serving items, food packages
  contain more than one serving. The first two
  lines on the approved food label tell you the
  size of a serving and the number of servings
  in the package.

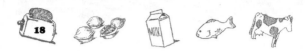

18

- Calorie content is the next important piece of data. The number of calories indicated is always per serving, not per package. You can determine the number of calories in the whole package by multiplying calories by number of servings. That's a good way to find out how many calories you are actually getting if you eat (or drink) "the whole thing!"
- The label tells you where the calories come from: the number of grams per serving of fat, protein, and carbohydrate.
- Because consumption of cholesterol, salt (sodium), and sugar are health concerns for many people, the grams per serving of those items are listed as well.
- Fiber, considered a health "plus," does not contribute any calories, but its presence is indicated for any foods that contain measurable amounts of it.

- The label also tells the percentage of certain nutrients' recommended daily value of each component, per serving. These percentages are based on a 2000-calorie diet, so your own daily allotment may differ.
- Ingredients are listed in order of their weight. That is, the earlier in the list an ingredient appears, the more (by weight) there is of it. This is where manufacturers may try to pull the wool over your eyes. But if you know their tricks, you won't be fooled.

The two areas where the label writers can fudge are sugar and fats:

Sugar is a carbohydrate, which means it contains 4 calories per gram. But if you look for sugar on the label and see it falls close to the bottom of the list, you might think there isn't much sugar in that particular food. In fact, sugar

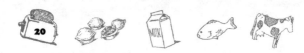

goes by many names, and most packaged foods contain more than one type of sugar. Among the masks sugar wears are: brown sugar, corn sweetener, corn syrup, fructose, fruit juice concentrate, glucose, dextrose, high-fructose corn syrup, honey, invert sugar, lactose, maltose, molasses, raw sugar, sucrose, and syrup.

Here's your secret weapon: Look at the part of the label that gives the total carbohydrate content. The number of grams of sugar is listed there. Then multiply the number of grams by 4 and you'll know the number of calories worth of sugar it contains.

Fat by any name contains 9 calories per gram. Again, small amounts (by weight) of many different fats can be used to hide the true story of the fat content. And again, the total fat content is given on the label. All you have to do is multiply the number of grams by 9 to find out the number of calories that come from fat.

Decoding Labeling Terms

Diet- and health-conscious people may look for the terms *low fat*, *reduced fat*, *no fat*, *low calorie*, *reduced calorie*, and *light* (or *lite*) when they are making food selections. But what do these terms mean? The short answer is that they do not necessarily mean a food is low in calories. The long answer comes from the FDA, which has set strict rules about the use of these terms:

- *Free* means that a product contains no amount of, or only trivial amounts of, fat, saturated fat, cholesterol, sodium, sugars, and/or calories.
- *Low* (or *Lo*) means the food can be eaten frequently without exceeding dietary guidelines for fat, saturated fat, cholesterol, sodium, and/or calories. According to this definition, low calorie means 40 calories or fewer per

serving; low-fat means 3 grams of fat or fewer per serving.

- *Reduced* means that the product contains at least 25 percent less of a nutrient or of calories than the regular product. However, a reduced claim can't be made on a product if the regular version meets the requirement for a "low" claim. For example, all pretzels are low in fat, so a particular brand of pretzels cannot be termed "reduced fat." And calling them low-fat does not make them low-calorie! Pretzels get their calories from carbohydrates, at the rate of 4 calories per gram.

- *Less* means that a food contains 25 percent less of a nutrient or of calories than the regular version. For example, pretzels that have 25 percent less fat than potato chips could carry a "less" claim.

- *Light* (or *Lite*) means that a product contains one-third fewer calories or half the fat of the regular version. If the food derives 50 percent or more of its calories from fat, the reduction must be 50 percent of the fat.

Be aware, though, that "light" can also be used to refer to salt (sodium) content and to describe such properties as texture and color, as long as the label explains the intent—for example, "light brown sugar" and "light and fluffy."

Rounding It All Up

All calorie counts in this book are rounded to the nearest 5. A few calories more or less do not make a big difference. These values have been calculated using a sample in a laboratory. What happens to a food when it enters your body

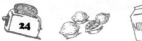

depends on many things besides its calorie content. Although we say that 3,500 calories equal a pound of stored body fat, that, too, is approximate. It depends on your metabolic rate, which varies among individuals and even within an individual, at any given time. It also depends upon your age, activity level, weight, and the ratio of body fat to muscle and bones.

Sources for calorie counts include the United States Department of Agriculture Nutrient Database for Standard Reference (Release 13, 1999), and the manufacturers' labels on selected products.

The federal government has two Web sites that are particularly useful for people interested in calories, and food and nutrition in general: *www.nutrition.gov* and *www.nalusda.gov.* Valuable information and links to other resources can be found at both of these sites.

Food	Serving Size	Calories
Alcoholic beverages*		
ale	12 oz	180
beer		
regular	12 oz	145
light	12 oz	100
low-alcohol (2.3% alcohol)	12 oz	75
non-alcoholic (less than .5% alcohol)	12 oz	65
malt liquor	12 oz	180
cider (6% alcohol)	12 oz	170
cocktails, mixed drinks**		
bloody mary	5 oz	115
brandy alexander	3 oz	270
daiquiri	2 oz	110
egg nog	3 oz	175
gimlet	3 oz	110
gin and tonic	6 oz	170
Irish coffee	6 oz	210
manhattan	2 oz	130
margarita	3½ oz	130
martini (gin or vodka)	2 oz	155
mint julep	4½ oz	190
piña colada	4½ oz	260
scotch and soda	4 oz	100

*Average calories; calorie counts vary widely among brands.

**Average calories as made from standard recipe; calorie counts for pre-mixed or bottled cocktail mixes vary among brands; calorie counts for all mixed drinks vary depending upon proof of alcohol used.

Beverages

Food	Serving Size	Calories

Alcoholic beverages (continued)

Food	Serving Size	Calories
screwdriver	7 oz	175
tequila sunrise	6 oz	200
tom collins	7½ oz	120
vodka and tonic (see *gin and tonic*)		
whiskey sour	3 oz	120
wine spritzer	6 oz	70

dessert wine

Food	Serving Size	Calories
madeira	2 oz	85
marsala	2 oz	110
port	2 oz	85
sherry, dry	2 oz	65
sherry, sweet	2 oz	85
vermouth, dry	2 oz	65
vermouth, sweet	2 oz	85

liqueurs

Food	Serving Size	Calories
amaretto	1 oz	75
brandy, fruit	1 oz	80
Benedictine	1 oz	90
Irish cream	1 oz	95
Cointreau	1 oz	100
coffee	1 oz	90
crème de cacao	1 oz	100
crème de menthe	1 oz	120
Drambuie	1 oz	105
Grand Marnier	1 oz	100
kirsch	1 oz	80
ouzo	1 oz	90
pastis	1 oz	90
Sambuca	1 oz	100

Food	Serving Size	Calories

Alcoholic beverages (continued)

liqueurs (continued)
Southern Comfort	1 oz	75
triple sec	1 oz	80

liquors: bourbon, brandy, gin, rum, scotch, tequila, vodka, whisky
80 proof	1 oz	65
86 proof	1 oz	70
90 proof	1 oz	75
100 proof	1 oz	80

table wine
champagne	4 oz	85
red	4 oz	80
rose	4 oz	80
white, dry	4 oz	75
white, sweet	4 oz	85

Breakfast Drinks*

chocolate
powder	individual packet	130
powder, sugar free	individual packet	70

strawberry
powder	individual packet	130
powder, sugar free	individual packet	70

vanilla
powder	individual packet	130

*Average calories; calorie counts vary widely among brands.

Food	Serving Size	Calories

Breakfast Drinks *(continued)*

vanilla *(continued)*

powder, sugar free	individual packet	70
ready to drink (all flavors)	10 oz	215

Chocolate Beverages*

chocolate drink, bottled	8 oz	124

cocoa, hot chocolate

with whole milk	8 oz	200
with nonfat milk	8 oz	140

cocoa, hot chocolate mix

with whole milk	8 oz	226
with 2% milk	8 oz	195
with water	8 oz	105
artificially sweetened	8 oz	50

Coffee

black
regular or decaffeinated

brewed or instant	8 oz	5

café au lait

with whole milk	8 oz	65
with nonfat milk	8 oz	45

caffe latte

with whole milk	8 oz	100

*Average calories; calorie counts vary widely among brands.

Beverages

Food	Serving Size	Calories

Coffee (continued)

caffe latte (continued)
with nonfat milk | 8 oz | 60

cappuccino
with whole milk | 8 oz | 70
with nonfat milk | 8 oz | 40

espresso | 2 oz | 4

flavored
made with water | 8 oz | 65
made with water, sugar free | 8 oz | 30

substitute, grain beverage | 8 oz | 10

Fruit Juices and Blends*

apple
juice, cider | 8 oz | 115
blended juice drink | 8 oz | 120

cranberry, cocktail
regular | 8 oz | 110
low-cal | 8 oz | 35

cranberry-apple | 8 oz | 125

cranberry-grape | 8 oz | 105

*Average calories; calorie counts vary widely among brands.

Beverages

Food	Serving Size	Calories
Fruit Juices and Blends *(continued)*		
fruit punch		
canned	8 oz	115
made from frozen concentrate	8 oz	115
made from powder	8 oz	95
grape		
canned/bottled	8 oz	155
juice drink, canned	8 oz	125
grapefruit		
fresh, canned, unsweetened	8 oz	95
fresh, canned, sweetened	8 oz	115
frozen	8 oz	100
lemon		
fresh	1 tbsp	4
	1 cup	60
concentrate	1 tbsp	3
	1 cup	48
lemonade		
made from frozen concentrate	8 oz	96
made from powder	8 oz	105
sugar free	8 oz	5
lime *(see lemon)*		
limeade		
made from frozen concentrate	8 oz	100

Food	Serving Size	Calories
Fruit Juices and Blends *(continued)*		
nectars: apricot, peach, pear, papaya	8 oz	140
orange		
juice, canned, fresh, frozen	8 oz	110
blended drink	8 oz	95
powdered drink	8 oz	115
sugar free	8 oz	5
orange-grapefruit	8 oz	110
pineapple, canned, frozen	8 oz	135
pineapple-grapefruit	8 oz	120
prune	8 oz	180
smoothies		
fruit	8 oz	305
fruit and milk	8 oz	125
fruit and yogurt	8 oz	140
nutritional shakes *(see Diet and Health Foods)*		
Shakes		
chocolate	12 oz	430
malted	12 oz	515
vanilla	12 oz	375
malted	12 oz	460

Beverages

Food	Serving Size	Calories
Sodas and Soft Drinks*		
bitter lemon	8 oz	100
cherry	8 oz	120
citrus	8 oz	95
club	8 oz	0
cola		
regular	8 oz	100
cherry	8 oz	110
collins mixer	8 oz	90
cream	8 oz	125
diet (all brands, all flavors)**	8 oz	2
Dr. Pepper	8 oz	100
ginger ale	8 oz	85
cherry	8 oz	120
grape	8 oz	105
lemon/lime	8 oz	100

*Average calories; calorie counts vary widely among brands. Calorie counts are based on an 8-oz serving; many beverage containers hold more than one serving, so read the label.

**Average; depending on brand and container size, diet sodas range from 1 to 5 calories.

Beverages

Food	Serving Size	Calories
Sodas and Soft Drinks *(continued)*		
mineral water		
plain	8 oz	0
flavored	8 oz	0
orange	8 oz	120
piña colada	8 oz	100
quinine water (see *tonic*)		
root beer	8 oz	110
seltzer		
plain	8 oz	0
flavored	8 oz	0
Seven-Up	8 oz	95
tonic	8 oz	85
vanilla	8 oz	105

Beverages

Sports Drinks

There are many brands of "sports" and "energy" drinks and they come in various sizes. The calorie count varies widely among brands. Read the label of any drink you use and pay particular attention to the serving size, as a bottle may contain more than one serving.

Food	Serving Size	Calories
Tea		
regular or decaffeinated (brewed or instant, unsweetened)	8 oz	1
flavored	8 oz	5
herbal	8 oz	2
iced*		
brewed, unsweetened	8 oz	1
from powdered mix		
unsweetened/artificially sweetened	8 oz	2
sweetened	8 oz	90
bottled, canned		
artificially sweetened	8 oz	3
sweetened	8 oz	80
Vegetable Juices		
bloody mary mix	8 oz	40
carrot	8 oz	100
tomato	8 oz	50
tomato beef	8 oz	90
tomato clam	8 oz	110
tomato-vegetable blend	8 oz	50

Beverages

*Average calories; calorie counts vary widely among brands.

Food	Serving Size	Calories
Bread*		
bran	I oz slice	90
challah	I oz slice	85
corn (see *Muffins, Sweet Rolls, Sweet Breads*)		
cracked wheat	I oz slice	70
focaccia (see *Pizza*)		
French	2 oz slice	155
honey-wheat berry	I oz slice	70
Irish soda	I oz slice	175
Italian	2 oz slice	160
multigrain	I oz slice	70
oat bran	I oz slice	70
oatmeal	I oz slice	75
pita	I	165
whole wheat	I	170
potato	I oz slice	100

*Average calories; calorie counts vary widely among brands as does weight of slices.

Food	Serving Size	Calories
Bread (continued)		
pumpernickel	1 oz slice	80
raisin	1 oz slice	75
rye	1 oz slice	80
sourdough	1 oz slice	140
white, sandwich style	1 oz slice	65
	thin slice (.6 oz)	45
whole wheat	1 slice	65
bread crumbs	1 cup	425
breadsticks	1 piece	40
croutons	1 cup	120
stuffing, dry	1 cup	180

Buns, Rolls, and Biscuits*

bagel		
plain, onion, seeded	small, 2 oz	160
	medium, 3 oz	240
	large, 4 oz	320
cinnamon raisin	medium, 3 oz	270
egg	medium, 3 oz	230

*Average calories; calorie counts vary widely among brands as does weight of slices.

Food	Serving Size	Calories
Buns, Rolls, and Biscuits *(continued)*		
biscuit		
baking powder	1 oz	100
buttermilk	1 oz	100
crescent	1 oz	100
croissant	2 oz	230
dinner	1	100
english muffin		
plain	1	135
whole wheat	1	135
cinnamon raisin	1	150
sandwich size	1	190
French	1	105
hamburger	1	125
hoagie	1	150
hot dog	1	110
Italian	1	280
kaiser, with poppy seeds	1	165
sandwich, with sesame seeds	1	140

Food	Serving Size	Calories
Crackers*		
animal	11 pieces	126
cheese		
peanut butter sandwich	1 piece	34
mini	14 pieces	150
corn cakes	2 cakes	50
crispbread	1 piece	40
goldfish	55 pieces	140
graham	1 oz; 4 squares	120
low fat	1 oz; 4 squares	110
melba toast	1 piece	20
matzo	1 square	110
oat thins	18 crackers	140
oyster	23 crackers	60
rice cakes	1 piece	35
saltine	1 piece	15
fat free	1 piece	15
sesame	3 pieces	70

*Average calories; calorie counts vary widely among brands.

Food	Serving Size	Calories
Crackers *(continued)*		
shredded wheat	7 pieces	140
reduced fat	8 pieces	130
snack rounds	5 pieces	80
minis	48 pieces	160
soda	2 pieces	60
stone ground wheat	5 pieces	80
vegetable thins	14 pieces	160
water	5 pieces	70
wheat	5 pieces	70
wheat thins	16 pieces	140
reduced fat	18 pieces	120
zwieback	1 piece	35
Muffins and Quick Breads*		
banana nut		
bread	1 oz slice	105
muffin	2½" x 2¼" slice	150
toaster muffin	1.4 oz	135

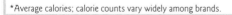

*Average calories; calorie counts vary widely among brands.

Breads, Crackers, and Baked Goods

Food	Serving Size	Calories
Muffins and Quick Breads *(continued)*		
blueberry muffin	2½" x 2¼"	160
toaster muffin	1.4 oz	135
Boston brown bread	1 slice	90
bran muffin	2 oz	185
carrot bread	2 oz slice	200
corn		
bread	2½" x 1½" piece	175
muffin	2½" x 2¼"	175
toaster muffin	1.4 oz	135
date nut bread	1 oz slice	80
hush puppy	1 piece	75
oat bran muffin	2 oz	155
scone	2 oz	200
shortcake	2 oz	220
Pizza*		
crust	1 lb; 12" diam	1200
cheese only	1 slice	235
	12" pie	1880

40

*Average calories; calorie counts vary widely among brands and recipes.

Food	Serving Size	Calories
Pizza (continued)		
pepperoni	1 slice	260
	12" pie	2080
sausage	1 slice	275
	12" pie	2200
mushroom	1 slice	240
	12" pie	1920
onion	1 slice	270
	12" pie	2160
focaccia	2 oz	200

Pancakes, Waffles, French Toast*

Food	Serving Size	Calories
pancake		
blueberry	4" cake	85
buckwheat	4" cake	60
buttermilk	4" cake	85
plain	4" cake	85
whole wheat	4" cake	90
waffles		
home made or mix	7" diam	220
frozen, toaster style	4" diam	85
french toast		
home recipe	1 slice	150
frozen	1 slice	125

*Average calories; calorie counts vary widely among brands, recipes, and restaurants.

Food	Serving Size	Calories
Taco and Tortilla Shells*		
burrito	12" diam	220
corn tortilla	7" diam	55
flour tortilla	8" diam	115
taco shell	5" diam	60
Wraps		
egg roll, raw	1 oz	80
lahvash	1 oz	100
wonton, raw	7" square	25

*Average calories; calorie counts vary widely among brands.

Food	Serving Size	Calories
Cereals*		
Alpha Bits	1 cup	130
Apple Jacks	1 cup	120
bran		
all bran	½ cup	80
extra fiber	½ cup	50
raisin nut	½ cup	200
flakes	1 oz	90
with raisins	1 oz	200
buds	1 oz	80
Cap'n Crunch	1 oz	105
Cheerios		
regular	1 cup	110
Apple Cinnamon	¾ cup	120
Honey Nut	1 cup	120
Multi-Grain	1 cup	110
Chex		
Corn	1 oz	110
Multi-Bran	2 oz	220
Rice	1 oz	110
Wheat	¾ cup	120
Cocoa Crispies	¾ cup	120
Cocoa Puffs	1 cup	120

*Average calories; calorie counts vary widely among brands.

Food	Serving Size	Calories
Cereals *(continued)*		
corn		
flakes	1 cup	100
frosted flakes	¾ cup	120
pops	1 cup	115
Count Chocula	1 cup	120
cream of rice, cooked	¾ cup	95
cream of wheat, cooked	¾ cup	100
Crispix	1 cup	110
Froot Loops	1 cup	120
Fruit and Fibre	1 cup	210
graham		
Cinnamon	¾ cup	120
Golden	¾ cup	120
granola	1 oz	130
Grape Nuts	½ cup	200
flakes	¾ cup	100
kasha, puffed	1 cup	70
Kix	1⅓ cup	120
Life	¾ cup	120

Food	Serving Size	Calories
Cereals (continued)		
muesli		
regular	½ cup	210
no sugar added	½ cup	200
multigrain flakes	¾ cup	110
oat bran	¾ cup	110
oatmeal (also see *Grains: oats*)		
regular, rolled, cooked	1 cup	145
instant, cooked	1 packet	105
instant, flavored, cooked	1 packet	150
rice		
crisps	1¼ cup	120
frosted	1 cup	105
puffed	1 cup	55
Special K	1 cup	110
Total	¾ cup	110
Trix	1 cup	120
wheat		
shredded	1 oz	100
mini	1 cup	170
mini, sugar coated	1 cup	200
flakes	1 cup	105
sugar coated	¾ cup	120
puffed	1 cup	50

Food	Serving Size	Calories

Cereals *(continued)*

Food	Serving Size	Calories
Wheatena, cooked	¾ cup	100
Wheaties	1 cup	110

Grains

barley		
uncooked	¼ cup	165
cooked	1 cup	195
buckwheat groats, roasted (kasha)		
uncooked	1 cup	400
cooked	1 cup	180
bulgur (see *wheat, cracked*)		
corn kernels (see *Snack Foods: Chips and Nibbles*)		
corn meal	1 cup	415
couscous		
uncooked	1 cup	680
cooked	1 cup	200
farina		
uncooked	1 oz	105
cooked	1 cup	115
flours (see *Sweets and Desserts: Baking Ingredients*)		

Food	Serving Size	Calories

Grains (continued)

grits (corn)
uncooked	¼ cup	140
cooked	1 cup	145

kasha (see *buckwheat groats*)

matzo meal	1 cup	440

millet
uncooked	1 oz	105
cooked	1 cup	285

oat bran
uncooked	½ cup	145
cooked	½ cup	45

oats
rolled, uncooked	½ cup	150
rolled, cooked	1 cup	145
steel cut, uncooked	⅓ cup	230

oatmeal (see *Cereals*)

polenta (see *cornmeal*)

quinoa, uncooked	½ cup	320

rye
whole grain	½ cup	320
flakes	⅓ cup	110

flour (see *Sweets and Desserts: Baking Ingredients*)

Cereals, Grains, Rice, and Pasta

Food	Serving Size	Calories
Grains *(continued)*		
tabbouleh (see *wheat, cracked*)		
tapioca, dry	⅓ cup	185
wheat		
berries, kernels	1 cup	215
bran	½ cup	65
cracked (bulgur, tabbouleh)		
uncooked	½ cup	240
cooked	1 cup	150
germ	¼ cup	110

Rice*

Food	Serving Size	Calories
arborio (see *white, short grain*)		
basmati (see *white, long grain*)		
brown		
uncooked	1 cup	700
cooked	1 cup	220
jasmine (see *white, long grain*)		
sushi (see *white, short grain*)		
white		
short grain		
uncooked	1 cup	720
cooked	1 cup	240

*For rice dishes, see *Soups, Stews, Casseroles, and Other Combination Foods.*

Food	Serving Size	Calories

Rice (continued)

white (continued)
long grain

uncooked	1 cup	670
cooked	1 cup	200

instant

uncooked	½ cup	370
cooked	½ cup	90

wild

uncooked	1 cup	570
cooked	1 cup	165

Pasta*

dry pasta (all shapes)

dry	2 oz	200
cooked	1 cup	200

fresh pasta

uncooked	4 oz	325
cooked	1 cup	190

filled pasta
ravioli

meat	3 oz; 1 cup	330
cheese	3 oz; 1 cup	290
tortellini	3 oz; ¾ cup	260

*For pasta dishes, see Soups, Stews, Casseroles, and Other Combination Foods.

Pasta *(continued)*

macaroni

Food	Serving Size	Calories
dry	2 oz	200
cooked	1 cup	200

noodles

Food	Serving Size	Calories
chow mein	1 cup	235
egg noodles		
dry	2 oz	220
cooked	1 cup	215
egg noodles, yolk free		
dry	2 oz	205
cooked	1 cup	205
rice (cellophane), dry	1 oz	100
soba (buckwheat)		
dry	1 oz	95
cooked	1 cup	100

Food	Serving Size	Calories

Milk

whole (3.5% fat)	8 oz	150
light, reduced fat (2% fat)	8 oz	120
low fat (1% fat)	8 oz	100
skim, fat free (0% fat)	8 oz	85
buttermilk, low fat (1% fat)	8 oz	100

chocolate milk

whole (3.5% fat)	8 oz	210
reduced fat (2% fat)	8 oz	200
low fat (1%)	8 oz	160

cocoa, chocolate drinks, and drink mixes (see *Beverages*)

condensed, sweetened

regular	2 tbsp	125
	1 cup	985
low fat	2 tbsp	120
	1 cup	960
fat free	2 tbsp	110
	1 cup	880

dry

whole, powder	1 cup	640
	1/4 cup	160
skim, nonfat, powder	1 cup	440
	1/4 cup	110
reconstituted	1 cup	80

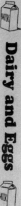

Dairy and Eggs

Food	Serving Size	Calories

Milk *(continued)*

evaporated

whole	1 cup	340
	2 tbsp	40
low fat (1% fat)	1 cup	200
	2 tbsp	25
skim, fat free (0% fat)	1 cup	200
	2 tbsp	25

rice (see *Diet and Health Foods: Milk Substitutes*)

soy (see *Diet and Health Foods: Milk Substitutes*)

Cream

crème fraîche	2 tbsp	110
half and half	1 cup	315
	1 oz	40
heavy	1 cup	820
	2 tbsp	105

ice cream (see *Sweets and Desserts*)

light	1 cup	470
	2 tbsp	60
mascarpone	1 oz	125

Dairy and Eggs

Food	Serving Size	Calories
Cream (continued)		
sour		
whole	I cup	495
	I tbsp	25
reduced fat	I cup	325
	I tbsp	20
fat free	I cup	160
	I tbsp	15
imitation	I cup	480
	I tbsp	60
sour cream dips (see *Snack Foods*)		
whipped*		
fresh	I cup	400
	I tbsp	25
pressurized	I cup	155
	I tbsp	10
nondairy topping		
regular, extra creamy	2 tbsp	25
light	2 tbsp	20
fat free	2 tbsp	15
powdered	2½ g	15
mix	2 tbsp	20
reconstituted with 2% milk	I cup	150

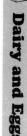

Dairy and Eggs

*Average calories; calorie counts vary widely among brands.

Food	Serving Size	Calories

Nondairy creamers*

liquid

regular	1 tbsp	20
flavored	1 tbsp	40
fat free	1 tbsp	10
flavored	1 tbsp	25
powdered	1 tsp	10

shakes
nutritional (see *Diet and Health Foods*)
smoothies (see *Beverages*)
thick, milk, malted (see *Sweets and Desserts*)

Yogurt*

plain

whole	8 oz container	180
low fat	8 oz container	145
nonfat	8 oz container	130

flavored (coffee, vanilla)

low fat	8 oz container	195
nonfat	8 oz container	190

with fruit

low fat	8 oz container	250
nonfat	8 oz container	240

frozen (see *Sweets and Desserts*)

Dairy and Eggs

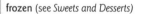

*Average calories; calorie counts vary widely among brands.

Food	Serving Size	Calories
Cheese*		
American		
regular	1 oz	105
	slice; 21 g	70
light, reduced fat	slice; 21 g	50
fat free	slice; 21 g	30
lactose free (nondairy)	slice; 19 g	25
Asiago	1 oz	100
blue (including Roquefort, Stilton, Gorgonzola, Danish)		
crumbled	1 oz	100
	1 cup	475
Boursin	1 oz	120
light	1 oz	45
brick	1 oz	105
Brie	1 oz	95
Camembert	1 oz	85
caraway	1 oz	110
Cheddar		
regular	1 oz	110
shredded	1 cup	450
low fat	1 oz	50
shredded	1 cup	200

*Average calories; calorie counts vary widely among brands.

Food	Serving Size	Calories

Cheese (continued)

cheese dip (see *Snack Foods*)

cheese food
| (prepared cheese product, Velveeta) | I oz | 90 |

cheese sauce (see *Extras: Sauces*)

cheese spread (American)
| | I oz | 85 |
| light | I oz | 65 |

chèvre (see *goat cheese*)

colby
regular	I oz	110
shredded	I cup	445
low fat	I oz	50
shredded	I cup	195

cottage cheese
plain, creamed (4% fat)	4 oz	115
plain, reduced fat (2% fat)	4 oz	100
plain, low fat (1% fat)	4 oz	80
plain, nonfat (0% fat)	4 oz	95
with fruit, creamed (4% fat)	4 oz	140
with fruit, low fat (1% fat)	4 oz	120
with fruit, nonfat (0% fat)	4 oz	110

cream cheese
regular	I oz	100
light, Neufchâtel	I oz	75
fat free	I oz	30

Dairy and Eggs

Food	Serving Size	Calories
Cheese *(continued)*		
cream cheese *(continued)*		
whipped	I tbsp	35
flavored	I tbsp	100
Edam	I oz	100
farmer	I oz	50
feta	I oz	75
crumbled	I cup	400
fondue	½ cup	245
fontina	I oz	110
gjetost	I oz	130
goat		
hard	I oz	130
soft	I oz	75
Gouda	I oz	100
Gruyère (see *Swiss*)		
Havarti	I oz	120
jack	I oz	105
Jarlsberg (see *Swiss*)		

Dairy and Eggs

Food	Serving Size	Calories
Cheese *(continued)*		
Limburger	1 oz	95
mozzarella		
whole milk	1 oz	80
shredded	1 cup	315
part skim	1 oz	70
shredded	1 oz	280
Muenster	1 oz	105
Neufchâtel (see *cream cheese*)		
Parmesan, grated	1 oz	130
	1 cup	460
Port Salut	1 oz	100
provolone	1 oz	100
ricotta		
whole milk	1 cup	430
part skim	1 cup	340
Romano	1 oz	110
string	1 oz	80
Swiss (Gruyère, Jarlsberg)	1 oz	110
Tilsit	1 oz	105
wine Cheddar spread	1 oz	95

Food	Serving Size	Calories
Eggs		
whole: raw, boiled, poached	large	80
	extra large	85
	jumbo	100
white	from 1 large egg	15
yolk	from 1 large egg	60
powdered		
whole	1 cup	505
	1 tbsp	30
white	1 cup	400
	1 tbsp	55
yolk	1 cup	445
	1 tbsp	30
deviled	1 whole	145
fried	1 large egg	90
omelet	2 large eggs	185
scrambled	1 large egg	100
egg nog (see *Beverages*)		
egg substitutes		
frozen	1 cup	385
liquid	1 cup	210
powder	.7 oz	90

Dairy and Eggs

Food	Serving Size	Calories

Diet Foods*
Nutritional Shakes

Boost	8 oz	240
Carnation Instant Breakfast		
regular, powder	1 envelope	130
no sugar added, powder	1 envelope	70
ready to drink	10 oz	220
Ensure		
regular	8 oz	250
plus	8 oz	355
Met-Rx, powder	2½ oz	260
Nutrament	1 can	200
Sweet Success, powder	1 scoop	90
Ultra Slim-Fast		
powder	1.2 oz	120
can	11 oz	220

Diet Bars

Boost	1 bar	190
Carnation Breakfast	1.27 oz bar	150

*For low-fat, reduced-fat, light, and sugar-free foods, see main categories for each.

Diet and Health Foods

Food	Serving Size	Calories

Diet Bars *(continued)*

Food	Serving Size	Calories
Figurine	2 bars	200
Met-RX	3½ oz bar	320
Nature Valley, low fat	1 oz bar	110
Nutrigrain	1⅓ oz bar	135
Sweet Rewards, fat free	1⅓ oz bar	120
Sweet Success	1 bar	114
Ultra Slim-Fast	1 oz bar	140

Diet Soft Drinks *(see Beverages)*

Sugar-Free Candy *(see Snack Foods)*

Health Foods

Food	Serving Size	Calories
brewer's yeast	1 oz	80
lecithin granules	1 tbsp	50

meat and poultry substitutes *(see Meat and Poultry)*

milk substitutes*		
rice milk	1 cup	150
soy milk		
regular	1 cup	140

*Average calories; calorie counts vary widely among brands.

Food	Serving Size	Calories

Health Foods *(continued)*

milk substitutes *(continued)*
soy milk *(continued)*

unsweetened	I cup	90
light	I cup	110
low fat	I cup	100
nonfat	I cup	80
seaweed, raw		
kelp	3½ oz	45
laver	3½ oz	35
spirulina	3½ oz	25
soy grits	I tbsp	30
tempeh	½ cup	165
tofu		
cake	I oz	20
cream (sour cream substitute)	2 tbsp	50
frozen dessert (see *Sweets and Desserts*)		
spread (cream cheese substitute)	I oz	80

Diet and Health Foods

Food	Serving Size	Calories
Dressings*		
bleu cheese		
regular	I tbsp	75
	I cup	1200
reduced fat	I tbsp	45
	I cup	720
made from mix	I tbsp	70
	I cup	1160
buttermilk		
ranch style	I tbsp	75
	I cup	1200
from mix	I tbsp	60
	I cup	960
caesar		
regular	I tbsp	65
	I cup	1050
reduced calorie	I tbsp	30
	I cup	480
made from mix	I tbsp	75
	I cup	1200
catalina		
regular	I tbsp	70
	I cup	1120
fat free	I tbsp	40
	I cup	640
cole slaw	I tbsp	75
	I cup	1200

*Average calories; calorie counts vary widely among brands and recipes.

Food	Serving Size	Calories
Dressings *(continued)*		
French (creamy)		
regular	1 tbsp	65
	1 cup	1040
reduced calorie	1 tbsp	25
	1 cup	400
fat free	1 tbsp	25
	1 cup	400
green goddess	1 tbsp	60
	1 cup	960
herb	1 tbsp	60
	1 cup	960
honey mustard		
regular or made from mix	1 tbsp	75
	1 cup	1200
fat free	1 tbsp	50
	1 cup	800
fat free, made from mix	1 tbsp	10
	1 cup	160
Italian		
regular and made from mix	1 tbsp	70
	1 cup	1120
reduced fat	1 tbsp	15
	1 cup	255
mayonnaise		
regular	1 tbsp	100
	1 cup	1575

Food	Serving Size	Calories

Dressings *(continued)*

mayonnaise *(continued)*

reduced fat, light	I tbsp	50
	I cup	800
fat free	I tbsp	10
	I cup	175

Miracle Whip

regular	I tbsp	70
	I cup	1120
light	I tbsp	40
	I cup	640
fat free	I tbsp	15
	I cup	240

ranch

regular	I tbsp	85
	I cup	1360
made from mix	I tbsp	60
	I cup	960
fat free	I tbsp	25
	I cup	400
reduced calorie, made from mix	I tbsp	30
	I cup	480

Russian

regular	I tbsp	75
	I cup	1200
reduced fat	I tbsp	25
	I cup	370

Food	Serving Size	Calories
Dressings (continued)		
thousand island		
regular	1 tbsp	60
	1 cup	960
reduced fat	1 tbsp	25
	1 cup	385
vinaigrette, oil and vinegar		
home recipe	1 tbsp	75
	1 cup	1200
regular	1 tbsp	55
	1 cup	880
fat free	1 tbsp	20
	1 cup	320
vinegar (see condiments)		
Gravy*		
au jus		
canned	2 tbsp	5
	1 cup	35
made from mix	2 tbsp	4
	1 cup	30
beef, canned	2 tbsp	15
	1 cup	100
brown		
canned	2 tbsp	15
	1 cup	115

*Average calories; calorie counts vary widely among brands and recipes.

Food	Serving Size	Calories
Gravy (continued)		
brown (continued)		
made from mix	2 tbsp	10
	1 cup	80
chicken		
canned	2 tbsp	20
	1 cup	170
made from mix	2 tbsp	10
	1 cup	90
cream	2 tbsp	15
	1 cup	135
mushroom		
canned	2 tbsp	10
	1 cup	85
made from mix	2 tbsp	8
	1 cup	70
onion		
canned	2 tbsp	10
	1 cup	95
made from mix	2 tbsp	10
	1 cup	80
pork		
canned	2 tbsp	20
	1 cup	145

Food	Serving Size	Calories
Gravy *(continued)*		
pork *(continued)*		
made from mix	2 tbsp	10
	1 cup	75
turkey		
canned	2 tbsp	10
	1 cup	90
made from mix	2 tbsp	10
	1 cup	90
Sauces*		
Alfredo	2 tbsp	90
	1 cup	720
black bean	1 tbsp	20
brown	2 tbsp	50
	1 cup	400
cheese	2 tbsp	60
	1 cup	480
clam		
red	2 tbsp	15
	1 cup	120
white	2 tbsp	40
	1 cup	300

*Average calories; calorie counts vary widely among brands and recipes.

Food	Serving Size	Calories
Sauces (continued)		
curry	2 tbsp	25
	1 cup	180
hollandaise	2 tbsp	85
	1 cup	340
mole poblano	2 tbsp	30
	1 cup	240
nacho cheese	2 tbsp	45
	1 cup	370
pesto	2 tbsp	75
	1 cup	630
pizza	2 tbsp	15
	1 cup	100
sloppy joe	¼ cup	50
	1 cup	200
teriyaki	2 tbsp	30
	1 cup	240
tomato		
homemade	2 tbsp	35
	1 cup	295
canned, jarred	2 tbsp	20
	1 cup	160

Food	Serving Size	Calories
Sauces (continued)		
white		
thin	2 tbsp	35
	1 cup	160
medium	2 tbsp	45
	1 cup	370
thick	2 tbsp	60
	1 cup	465

Condiments*

Food	Serving Size	Calories
barbecue sauce	1 tbsp	25
	1 cup	190
capers	1 tbsp	5
catsup (see *ketchup*)		
chili sauce	2 tbsp	30
	1 cup	240
chutney	2 tbsp	40
cocktail sauce (ketchup based)	2 tbsp	30
	1 cup	240
hoisin sauce	½ cup	180
horseradish	1 tbsp	0

*Average calories; calorie counts vary widely among brands and recipes.

Food	Serving Size	Calories
Condiments (continued)		
ketchup	1 tbsp	16
mustard		
American style	1 tbsp	4
French style	1 tbsp	5
honey	1 tbsp	10
relish		
sweet pickle	1 tbsp	20
hot dog	1 tbsp	15
remoulade	2 tbsp	110
salsa	2 tbsp	10
soy sauce	1 tbsp	10
steak sauce	1 tbsp	20
sweet and sour	2 tbsp	40
Tabasco	1 tsp	1
taco sauce	1 tbsp	5
tartar sauce		
regular	2 tbsp	100
nonfat	2 tbsp	25
vinegar		
balsamic, red wine, flavored, herb	1 tbsp	2

Food	Serving Size	Calories
Condiments (continued)		
vinegar (continued)		
cider, white	I tbsp	5
Worcestershire sauce	I tbsp	5
Flavorings		
Accent	I tsp	0
adobo	I tsp	0
bitters	½ tsp	2
bouillon cubes	I cube	5
broth powder	I tsp	5
butter flavoring	I tsp	5
extracts		
almond	I tsp	10
orange	I tsp	20
mint	I tsp	20
vanilla	I tsp	10
miso	I tbsp	35
	I cup	565
Herbs and Spices		
allspice, ground	I tsp	5

Food	Serving Size	Calories
Herbs and Spices *(continued)*		
anise seed	I tsp	5
basil		
fresh	2 tbsp	0
dried	I tsp	5
bay leaf	I leaf	5
caraway seed	I tsp	7
celery seed	I tsp	10
chervil, dried	I tsp	0
chili powder	I tsp	10
Chinese parsley (see *coriander*)		
chives		
fresh, chopped	I tbsp	0
dried, freeze dried	¼ tsp	0
cilantro (see *coriander*)		
cinnamon, ground	I tsp	5
cloves, ground	I tsp	5
coriander (cilantro, Chinese parsley)		
fresh leaf	¼ cup	0
dried leaf	I tsp	5

Food	Serving Size	Calories
Herbs and Spices *(continued)*		
coriander (cilantro, Chinese parsley) *(continued)*		
seed	1 tsp	5
cumin		
ground	1 tsp	5
seed	1 tsp	5
curry powder	1 tsp	5
dill		
seed	1 tsp	5
weed, fresh	1 cup	5
weed, dried	1 tsp	5
fennel seed	1 tsp	5
garlic (see *Vegetables*)		
garlic powder	1 tsp	10
ginger		
fresh root	¼ cup	15
ground	1 tsp	5
mace	1 tsp	10
marjoram, dried	1 tsp	5
mustard		
powder	1 tsp	10
seed	1 tsp	15

Food	Serving Size	Calories
Herbs and Spices *(continued)*		
nutmeg, ground	1 tsp	10
onion powder	1 tsp	5
oregano, dried	1 tsp	5
paprika	1 tsp	5
parsley fresh dried	 ½ cup 1 tsp	 10 5
pepper, ground black, red, white	1 tsp	5
poppy seed	1 tsp	15
poultry seasoning	1 tsp	5
rosemary, dried	1 tsp	5
saffron	1 tsp	5
sage, dried, rubbed	1 tsp	5
salt and **salt substitutes**	1 tsp	0
savory, ground	1 tsp	5
shallots (see *Vegetables*)		
tarragon, dried	1 tsp	5

Food	Serving Size	Calories
Herbs and Spices *(continued)*		
thyme		
fresh	I tsp	0
dried	I tsp	5
turmeric, ground	I tsp	5

Food	Serving Size	Calories
Fats		
butter		
salted or unsalted	I tbsp	110
	I stick; ¼ lb; ½ cup	880
whipped	I tbsp	65
	I cup	1080
light (margarine/butter blend)	I tbsp	105
	I stick; ¼ lb; ½ cup	815
margarine		
regular	I tbsp	100
	I stick; ¼ lb; ½ cup	815
soft (tub)	I tbsp	100
	I cup	1625
liquid	I tbsp	50
	I cup	800
substitutes		
Benecol	I tbsp	80
Brummel & Brown	I tbsp	45
I Can't Believe It's Not Butter	I tbsp	90
light	I tbsp	50
Olivio	I tbsp	80
Smart Balance	I tbsp	80
Smartbeat	I tbsp	20
Take Control	I tbsp	50
light	I tbsp	40
chicken fat	I tbsp	115
	I cup	1850
duck fat (see *chicken fat*)		

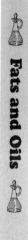

Food	Serving Size	Calories
Fats (continued)		
goose fat (see *chicken fat*)		
lard	I tbsp	115
	I cup	1850
salt pork	I oz	210
shortening (solid)		
vegetable oil	I tbsp	113
	I cup	1812
vegetable oil/lard blend	I tbsp	115
	I cup	1845
suet (beef)	I oz	240
tallow (beef, mutton)	I tbsp	115
	I cup	1850
turkey fat (see *chicken fat*)		
Oils		
canola (rapeseed)	I tbsp	125
	I cup	1925
cocoa butter	I tbsp	120
	I cup	1925
coconut	I tbsp	115
	I cup	1880

Food	Serving Size	Calories
Oils *(continued)*		
cod liver (see *fish oil*)		
corn	I tbsp	120
	I cup	1925
cottonseed	I tbsp	120
	I cup	1925
fish oil (cod liver, herring, menhaden, salmon)	I tbsp	125
grapeseed	I tbsp	120
	I cup	1925
olive	I tbsp	120
	I cup	1910
nut (almond, apricot kernel, hazelnut, walnut)	I tbsp	125
	I cup	2000
palm	I tbsp	120
	I cup	1910
peanut	I tbsp	120
	I cup	1910
safflower	I tbsp	120
	I cup	1925

Fats and Oils

Food	Serving Size	Calories
Oils *(continued)*		
sesame	1 tbsp	120
	1 cup	1925
soybean	1 tbsp	120
	1 cup	1925
spray	1 spray	2
sunflower	1 tbsp	120
	1 cup	1925
vegetable (blended)	1 tbsp	120
	1 cup	1925
wheat germ	1 tbsp	120
	1 cup	1925

Food	Serving Size	Calories

Note: Edible portion only; no bones or shells.

abalone

raw	3 oz	90
fried	3 oz	160

anchovy

raw, free	3 oz	110
canned, in oil	5 filets	40
paste	1 tsp	14

bass

black

raw	4 oz	105
steamed, poached, broiled, grilled, baked, microwaved	3½ oz	105
sautéed	3½ oz	125

Chilean sea bass (see *grouper*)

striped

raw	4 oz	110
steamed, poached, broiled, grilled, baked, microwaved	3½ oz	110
sautéed	3½ oz	130

blackfish (see *tautog*)

bluefish

raw	4 oz	140
steamed, poached, broiled, grilled, baked, microwaved	3½ oz	140

Food	Serving Size	Calories
butterfish		
raw	4 oz	165
sautéed	3½ oz	185
calamari (squid)		
raw	4 oz	105
grilled	3½ oz	105
fried	3 oz	150
carp		
raw	4 oz	145
poached	3½ oz	145
fried, sautéed	3½ oz	165
catfish		
raw	4 oz	150
broiled	3½ oz	150
fried, breaded	4 oz	227
caviar, black or red	1 tbsp	40
clams		
raw	3 oz	65
steamed	3 oz	125
fried, breaded	4 oz	170
canned, drained	3 oz	125
clam juice	1 cup	5
cod		
raw	4 oz	95

Food	Serving Size	Calories
cod (continued)		
steamed, poached, broiled, baked, microwaved	3½ oz	105
sautéed	3½ oz	125
salt (dried)	3 oz	245
crab		
Alaska king, steamed or boiled	3 oz	80
blue, steamed or boiled	3 oz	85
Dungeness, steamed or boiled	3 oz	95
legs, imitation (see *surimi*)		
crayfish, boiled	3 oz	75
croaker		
raw	4 oz	115
fried, breaded	4 oz	220
dolphin fish (see *mahi-mahi*)		
dover sole (see *flounder*)		
eel		
raw	4 oz	210
grilled, poached, microwaved	3½ oz	235
smoked	3 oz	285
finnan haddie (see *haddock, smoked*)		
fish filets, frozen		
battered	4 oz	300
lightly battered	3⅓ oz	200

Food	Serving Size	Calories
fish sticks, frozen	3 oz	200
flounder		
raw	4 oz	100
grilled, poached, microwaved	3½ oz	100
fried, breaded	4 oz	240
gefilte fish		
regular	2 oz	55
with jelled broth	2 oz	80
sweet	2 oz	65
with jelled broth	2 oz	95
grouper (rock cod, Chilean sea bass)		
raw	4 oz	105
steamed, poached, broiled,		
grilled, baked, microwaved	3½ oz	105
sautéed	3½ oz	125
fried, breaded	3½ oz	200
haddock		
raw	4 oz	100
steamed, poached, broiled,		
baked, grilled, microwaved	3½ oz	110
sautéed	3½ oz	185
smoked (finnan haddie)	3 oz	100
hake (see *whiting*)		
halibut		
raw	4 oz	125

Food	Serving Size	Calories
halibut *(continued)*		
steamed, poached, broiled,		
grilled, baked, microwaved	3½ oz	135
sautéed	3½ oz	220
herring		
raw	4 oz	175
grilled, broiled	3½ oz	200
pickled	1 oz	60
in sour cream	1 oz	50
smoked (kippered)	2 oz	125
canned	2 oz	120
with tomato sauce	2 oz	100
kingfish (see *mackerel*)		
ling		
raw	4 oz	100
steamed, poached, broiled,		
baked, microwaved	3½ oz	110
sautéed	3½ oz	180
fried, breaded	4 oz	200
lobster		
raw	4 oz	105
boiled, steamed, broiled, baked	3 oz	90
lox (see *salmon, smoked*)		
mackerel		
raw	4 oz	160
grilled, broiled	3½ oz	160

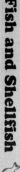

Fish and Shellfish

Food	Serving Size	Calories
mahi-mahi (dolphin fish)		
raw	4 oz	100
steamed, poached, broiled, baked, grilled, microwaved	3½ oz	110
sautéed	3½ oz	180
mako (see *shark*)		
monkfish (lotte)		
raw	4 oz	85
steamed, poached, broiled, baked, grilled, microwaved	3½ oz	95
sautéed	3½ oz	180
mullet		
raw	4 oz	135
sautéed	3½ oz	210
fried, breaded	4 oz	250
mussels		
raw	4 oz	100
steamed	4 oz	200
Nova Scotia (see *salmon, smoked*)		
octopus		
raw	4 oz	95
boiled	3½ oz	160
orange roughy		
raw	4 oz	80

Food	Serving Size	Calories
orange roughy *(continued)*		
steamed, poached, broiled, baked, microwaved	3½ oz	90
sautéed	3½ oz	175
oysters		
raw	3 oz; 6 medium	55
fried, breaded	3 oz; 6 medium	170
Rockefeller	6	440
perch		
raw	4 oz	100
steamed, poached, broiled, baked, microwaved	3½ oz	115
sautéed	3½ oz	200
fried, breaded	4 oz	240
pike (pickerel)		
raw	4 oz	115
sautéed	3½ oz	180
fried, breaded	4 oz	200
plaice (see *flounder*)		
pollack		
raw	4 oz	105
steamed, poached, broiled, baked, microwaved	3½ oz	115
sautéed	3½ oz	200
pompano (yellowtail)		
raw	4 oz	185

Food	Serving Size	Calories
pompano (yellowtail) *(continued)*		
grilled, poached, microwaved	3½ oz	210
sautéed	3½ oz	300
porgy		
raw	4 oz	130
poached, broiled, microwaved	3½ oz	135
sautéed	3½ oz	210
fried, breaded	4 oz	230
rockfish (see *bass, striped*)		
sable, smoked	3 oz	220
salmon (pink)		
raw	4 oz	135
steamed, poached, broiled, baked, grilled, microwaved	3½ oz	150
sautéed	3½ oz	220
canned	3 oz	120
salmon (red)		
raw	4 oz	190
steamed, poached, broiled, baked, grilled, microwaved	3½ oz	215
sautéed	3½ oz	300
canned	3 oz	150
smoked (lox, Nova Scotia, Scotch)	3 oz	100
scallops		
raw	3 oz	75

Food	Serving Size	Calories
scallops *(continued)*		
poached, steamed, baked,		
grilled, broiled, microwaved	3 oz	100
sautéed	3 oz	180
fried, breaded	3 oz	200
scrod (see *haddock*)		
scup (see *porgy*)		
shad		
raw	4 oz	225
broiled	3½ oz	250
sautéed	3½ oz	320
roe		
raw	3 oz	120
sautéed	3 oz	200
shark (mako)		
raw	4 oz	150
grilled, broiled, poached	3½ oz	160
sautéed	3½ oz	250
shrimp		
raw	3 oz; 12 large	90
poached, boiled, steamed, baked,		
grilled, broiled, microwaved	3 oz; 15 large	84
sautéed	3 oz; 12 large	175
fried, breaded	3 oz; 11 large	205
skate (ray)		
raw	4 oz	110

Food	Serving Size	Calories
skate (ray) *(continued)*		
poached	3½ oz	110
sautéed	3½ oz	200
smelt		
raw	4 oz	115
broiled	3½ oz	120
sautéed	3½ oz	200
fried, breaded	4 oz	225
snapper		
raw	4 oz	115
poached, boiled, steamed, baked, microwaved, grilled, broiled	3½ oz	125
sautéed	3½ oz	210
fried, breaded	4 oz	225
sole (see *flounder*)		
squid (see *calamari*)		
sturgeon		
raw	4 oz	120
grilled, baked, poached, microwaved	3½ oz	115
smoked	3 oz	145
surimi (imitation crab legs)	3 oz	85
swordfish		
raw	4 oz	135
grilled, broiled, poached, baked, microwaved	3½ oz	155

Food	Serving Size	Calories
swordfish *(continued)*		
sautéed	3½ oz	225
tautog (blackfish)		
raw	4 oz	100
grilled, broiled, poached,		
baked, microwaved	3½ oz	115
sautéed	3½ oz	200
tilefish		
raw	4 oz	110
poached, boiled, steamed,		
baked, broiled, microwaved	3½ oz	145
sautéed	3½ oz	200
trout		
brook, rainbow		
raw	4 oz	155
poached, steamed, microwaved,		
baked, broiled, grilled	3½ oz	170
sautéed	3½ oz	250
sea (weakfish)		
raw	4 oz	115
poached, steamed, microwaved,		
baked, broiled, grilled	3½ oz	130
sautéed	3½ oz	200
tuna		
albacore, bluefin		
raw	4 oz	165
grilled, broiled, baked, microwaved	3½ oz	180
sautéed	3½ oz	250

Food	Serving Size	Calories
tuna *(continued)*		
yellowfin, skipjack		
raw	4 oz	120
grilled, broiled, baked, microwaved	3½ oz	140
sautéed	3½ oz	210
canned		
light, in water	3 oz	110
light, in oil, drained	3 oz	170
white, in water	3 oz	100
white, in oil, drained	3 oz	160
turbot		
raw	4 oz	110
poached, broiled, microwaved	3½ oz	120
sautéed	3½ oz	200
whitefish		
raw	4 oz	150
poached, broiled, microwaved	3½ oz	170
sautéed	3½ oz	250
smoked	3 oz	90
whiting (hake)		
raw	4 oz	100
poached, baked, microwaved	3½ oz	115
sautéed	3½ oz	200
fried, breaded	4 oz	300
yellowtail (see *pompano*)		

Food	Serving Size	Calories

Note: For fruit juices, see *Beverages;* for fruit pies and jams, jellies, preserves, and spreads, see *Sweets and Desserts.*

apple

whole, raw, with skin	small; 4 oz	65
	medium; 5 oz	85
	large; 7½ oz	125
cooked, without skin	1 cup	90
canned, sweetened, drained	1 cup	135
caramel-covered	1 medium	170
dried	1 cup	210

apple butter (see *Sweets and Desserts*)

apple pie (see *Sweets and Desserts*)

apple sauce

regular	1 cup	195
unsweetened, sugar free	1 cup	105

apricot

whole, raw	small; 1¼ oz	15
	medium; 2 oz	25
	large; 3 oz	35
candied	1 oz	100
canned		
in water	1 cup	65
in light syrup	1 cup	160
in heavy syrup	1 cup	210
dried	1 cup	380
	½ fruit	10

Fruits

Food	Serving Size	Calories
banana		
fresh	small; 4 oz, with skin	55
	medium; 5 oz, with skin	80
	large; 7 oz, with skin	105
mashed	1 cup	205
sliced	1 cup	140
dried	1 cup	345
blackberries		
fresh	1 cup	75
canned, in heavy syrup	1 cup	235
frozen, unsweetened	1 cup	95
blueberries		
fresh	1 cup	80
	1 pint	225
canned, in heavy syrup	1 cup	225
frozen		
unsweetened	1 cup	80
sweetened	1 cup	185
boysenberries		
canned in heavy syrup	1 cup	225
cantaloupe		
slice	2 oz, without skin	15
pieces	1 cup	145
casaba melon		
slice	6 oz, without skin	45
pieces	1 cup	45

Food	Serving Size	Calories
cherries		
sour	I cherry	5
	I lb	200
canned		
in light syrup	I cup	190
in heavy syrup	I cup	235
sweet	I cherry	5
	I lb	290
canned		
in water	I cup	115
in light syrup	I cup	170
in heavy syrup	I cup	210
citrus peel		
fresh	I tbsp	5
candied	I oz	90
cranberries		
fresh, raw	I cup	45
jelly	I cup	420
whole fruit sauce	I cup	440
dried	½ cup	180
currants		
fresh	I cup	65
dried	I cup	410
dates		
fresh or dried	I date	25
pitted, chopped	I cup	490

Food	Serving Size	Calories
figs		
fresh	large; 2½" diam	45
	medium; 2¼" diam	35
	small; 1½" diam	30
canned		
in water	1 cup	15
in light syrup	1 cup	20
in heavy syrup	1 cup	25
dried	1 fig	50
fruit leather (see *Snack Foods: Candy*)		
fruit salad (fruit cocktail), canned		
in water	1 cup	75
in light syrup	1 cup	140
in heavy syrup	1 cup	180
ginger (see *Extras: Herbs and Spices*)		
granadilla (see *passionfruit*)		
grapefruit	½ large; 4½" diam	55
sections and juice	1 cup	75
canned, in light syrup	1 cup	150
grapes	1 grape	15
	1 cup	115
guava	1 cup	85

Fruits

Food	Serving Size	Calories
honeydew		
slice	3½ oz	45
pieces	1 cup	60
kiwi	1 fruit	45
kumquat, fresh	1 fruit	10
lemon	1 fruit	20
lime	1 fruit	20
mandarin		
fresh	1 large	45
canned, in light syrup	1 cup	155
mango		
fresh, flesh only	1 cup, slices	110
dried	1 oz	100
nectarine	1 fruit; 2½" diam	70
orange		
whole, fresh	small; 2½" diam	45
	large; 3" diam	85
sections, fresh	1 cup	85
papaya	1 cup, cubes	55
passionfruit (granadilla)	1 fruit	120
	1 cup, cubes	230

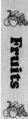

Fruits

Food	Serving Size	Calories
peach		
fresh, whole	large; 6½ oz	70
	small; 4 oz	40
canned		
in water	1 cup	60
in light syrup	1 cup	135
in heavy syrup	1 cup	195
pear		
fresh, whole, all types	large; 8 oz	125
	small; 6 oz	100
canned		
in water	1 cup	70
in light syrup	1 cup	145
in heavy syrup	1 cup	200
dried	1 cup	475
	½ pear	50
persimmon		
Japanese, large	1 fruit	120
American, small	1 fruit	32
pineapple		
fresh, flesh only		
slice	⅛ pineapple	60
diced	1 cup	75
canned		
in water	1 cup	80
	1 slice	15
in light syrup	1 cup	130
	1 slice	25

Fruits

Food	Serving Size	Calories
pineapple *(continued)*		
canned *(continued)*		
in heavy syrup	I cup	200
	I slice	40
dried	I oz	70
plantain		
raw	I cup	180
cooked	I cup	180
plum		
damson	½ oz	8
all other types	2 oz	35
canned, purple		
in water	I cup	100
in light syrup	I cup	160
in heavy syrup	I cup	230
pomegranate	I fruit	105
prickly pear	I fruit	40
prune		
dried, pitted	I fruit	20
	I cup	450
stewed	I cup	315
canned, in heavy syrup	I cup	245
quince	I fruit	50
raisins	I cup; 5 oz	435

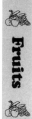

Food	Serving Size	Calories
raspberries		
fresh, whole	10 berries	10
	1 cup	60
	1 pint	150
frozen, sweetened	1 cup	260
strawberries		
fresh	1 berry	5
halves	1 cup	45
purée, unsweetened	1 cup	50
frozen		
whole, unsweetened	1 cup	75
sliced, sweetened	1 cup	245
tangerine	1 fruit	45
watermelon		
slice	4 oz	10
cubes	1 cup	50

Fruits

Food	Serving Size	Calories

Note: Edible portion, cooked as indicated, fat trim as indicated. Listings are for representative samples; calorie counts are approximate since degree of marbling (fat within meat) and trimming of surrounding fat, cooking temperature, and doneness vary.

Meat: Beef

bologna (see *Luncheon and Deli Meats*)

brain (see *Organ Meats*)

brisket
whole, braised, lean and fat	3½ oz; ¼" fat trim	405
whole, braised, lean	3½ oz; 0" fat trim	220

chuck roast (pot roast)
choice, braised, lean and fat	3½ oz; ¼" fat trim	350
choice, braised, lean	3½ oz; 0" fat trim	220
select, braised, lean and fat	3½ oz; ¼" fat trim	315
select, braised, lean	3½ oz; 0" fat trim	200

corned beef, cooked   3½ oz   250

frankfurter (see *Luncheon and Deli Meats*)

flank
braised, lean and fat	3½ oz; 0" fat trim	265
braised, lean	3½ oz; 0" fat trim	235
broiled, lean and fat	3½ oz; 0" fat trim	225
broiled, lean	3½ oz; 0" fat trim	205

Meat and Poultry

Meat: Beef *(continued)*

ground
regular fat

baked, medium-well	3½ oz	300
broiled, medium-well	3½ oz	290
pan fried, medium-well	3½ oz	295

lean

baked, medium-well	3½ oz	280
broiled, medium-well	3½ oz	275
pan fried, medium-well	3½ oz	275

heart (see *Organ Meats*)

hot dog (see *Luncheon and Deli Meats: frankfurter*)

kidney (see *Organ Meats*)

liver (see *Organ Meats*)

loin
porterhouse steak

broiled, lean and fat	3½ oz; ¼" fat trim	225
broiled, lean	3½ oz; ¼" fat trim	215

T-bone steak

broiled, lean and fat	3½ oz; ¼" fat trim	310
broiled, lean	3½ oz; ¼" fat trim	205

tenderloin

choice, broiled, lean and fat	3½ oz; ¼" fat trim	305
choice, broiled, lean	3½ oz; ¼" fat trim	220
prime, broiled, lean and fat	3½ oz; ¼" fat trim	315
prime, broiled, lean	3½ oz; ¼" fat trim	230

Meat and Poultry

Food	Serving Size	Calories

Meat: Beef (continued)

loin (continued)
top sirloin steak

choice, broiled, lean and fat	3½ oz; ¼" fat trim	270
choice, broiled, lean	3½ oz; 0" fat trim	200
select, broiled, lean and fat	3½ oz; ¼" fat trim	245
select, broiled, lean	3½ oz; 0" fat trim	180

lung (see *Organ Meats*)

pancreas (see *Organ Meats*)

rib

whole, choice, roasted, lean and fat	3½ oz; ¼" fat trim	390
whole, choice, roasted, lean	3½ oz; ¼" fat trim	245
whole, prime, roasted, lean and fat	3½ oz; ¼" fat trim	410
whole, prime, roasted, lean	3½ oz; ¼" fat trim	290

round

bottom, choice, braised, lean and fat	3½ oz; ¼" fat trim	285
bottom, choice, braised, lean	3½ oz; 0" fat trim	215
bottom, select, braised, lean and fat	3½ oz; ¼" fat trim	260
bottom, select, braised, lean	3½ oz; 0" fat trim	195
bottom, choice, roasted, lean and fat	3½ oz; ¼" fat trim	260
bottom, choice, roasted, lean	3½ oz; 0" fat trim	195
bottom, select, roasted, lean and fat	3½ oz; ¼" fat trim	235
bottom, select, roasted, lean	3½ oz; 0" fat trim	170
eye, choice, roasted, lean and fat	3½ oz; ¼" fat trim	240
eye, choice, roasted, lean	3½ oz; 0" fat trim	175
eye, select, roasted, lean and fat	3½ oz; ¼" fat trim	215
eye, select, roasted, lean	3½ oz; 0" fat trim	155

Food	Serving Size	Calories
Meat: Beef (continued)		
round (continued)		
full cut (steak), choice, broiled, lean and fat	3½ oz; ¼" fat trim	240
full cut (steak), choice, broiled, lean	3½ oz; ¼" fat trim	190
full cut (steak), select, broiled, lean and fat	3½ oz; ¼" fat trim	225
full cut (steak), select, broiled, lean	3½ oz; ¼" fat trim	170
tip, choice, roasted, lean and fat	3½ oz; ¼" fat trim	245
tip, choice, roasted, lean	3½ oz; 0" fat trim	180
tip, prime, roasted, lean and fat	3½ oz; ¼" fat trim	275
tip, prime, roasted, lean	3½ oz; ¼" fat trim	215
top, choice, braised, lean and fat	3½ oz; ¼" fat trim	260
top, choice, braised, lean	3½ oz; 0" fat trim	205
top, select, braised, lean and fat	3½ oz; ¼" fat trim	235
top, select, braised, lean	3½ oz; 0" fat trim	190
top, choice, broiled, lean and fat	3½ oz; ¼" fat trim	225
top, choice, broiled, lean	3½ oz; ¼" fat trim	190
top, prime, broiled, lean and fat	3½ oz; ¼" fat trim	230
top, prime, broiled, lean	3½ oz; ¼" fat trim	215
salami (see *Luncheon and Deli Meats*)		
shank		
choice, simmered, lean and fat	3½ oz; ¼" fat trim	265
choice, simmered, lean	3½ oz; ¼" fat trim	200
short ribs		
braised, lean and fat	3½ oz	470
braised, lean	3½ oz	295
spleen (see *Organ Meats*)		

Food	Serving Size	Calories

Meat: Beef *(continued)*

sweetbreads (see *Organ Meats*)

tongue (see *Organ Meats*)

tripe (see *Organ Meats*)

Meat: Lamb

brain (see *Organ Meats*)

cubes		
braised, lean	3½ oz	225
broiled, lean	3½ oz	185
ground, broiled	3½ oz	285

heart (see *Organ Meats*)

kidney (see *Organ Meats*)

leg		
roasted, lean and fat	3½ oz	260
roasted, lean	3½ oz	190

liver (see *Organ Meats*)

loin		
chop, broiled, lean and fat	3½ oz	315
chop, broiled, lean	3½ oz	215
roasted, lean and fat	3½ oz	310
roasted, lean	3½ oz	200

Food	Serving Size	Calories

Meat: Lamb *(continued)*

lung (see *Organ Meats*)

pancreas (see *Organ Meats*)

rib

chop, broiled, lean and fat	3½ oz	260
chop, broiled, lean	3½ oz	235
roasted, lean and fat	3½ oz	360
roasted, lean	3½ oz	230

shank

braised, lean and fat	3½ oz	245
braised, lean	3½ oz	185

shoulder

braised, lean and fat	3½ oz	345
braised, lean	3½ oz	285
chop, broiled, lean and fat	3½ oz	280
chop, broiled, lean	3½ oz	210
roasted, lean and fat	3½ oz	275
roasted, lean	3½ oz	205

spleen (see *Organ Meats*)

tongue (see *Organ Meats*)

Meat: Organ Meats

belly, pork, raw	1 oz	145

Food	Serving Size	Calories
Meat: Organ Meats *(continued)*		
brain		
beef, pan fried	3½ oz	195
beef, simmered	3½ oz	160
lamb, braised	3½ oz	145
lamb, pan fried	3½ oz	275
pork, braised	3½ oz	140
veal, braised	3½ oz	135
veal, pan fried	3½ oz	215
chitterlings, pork, simmered	3½ oz	305
ear, pork	4 oz; 1 ear	185
feet, pork		
pickled	3½ oz	205
simmered	3½ oz	195
smoked hock	3½ oz	200
heart		
beef, simmered	3½ oz	175
lamb, braised	3½ oz	185
pork, braised	4½ oz; 1 heart	190
veal, braised	3½ oz	185
jowl, pork, raw	3½ oz	655
kidney		
beef, simmered	3½ oz	145
lamb, braised	3½ oz	135
pork, braised	3½ oz	150
veal, braised	3½ oz	165

Food	Serving Size	Calories
Meat: Organ Meats *(continued)*		
liver		
beef, braised	3½ oz	160
beef, pan fried	3½ oz	215
lamb, braised	3½ oz	220
lamb, pan fried	3½ oz	240
pork, braised	3½ oz	165
veal (calf), braised	3½ oz	165
veal (calf), pan fried	3½ oz	245
lung		
beef, braised	3½ oz	120
lamb, braised	3½ oz	115
pork, braised	3½ oz	100
veal, braised	3½ oz	105
pancreas		
beef, braised	3½ oz	270
lamb, braised	3½ oz	235
pork, braised	3½ oz	220
veal, braised	3½ oz	255
scrapple	1 oz	60
spleen		
beef, braised	3½ oz	145
lamb, braised	3½ oz	155
pork, braised	3½ oz	150
veal, braised	3½ oz	130
stomach, pork, raw	3½ oz	155

Food	Serving Size	Calories

Meat: Organ Meats *(continued)*

sweetbread (thymus)

beef, braised	3½ oz	320
veal, braised	3½ oz	175
tail, pork, simmered	3½ oz	395

tongue

beef, simmered	3½ oz	285
lamb, braised	3½ oz	275
pork, braised	3½ oz	270
veal, braised	3½ oz	200
tripe, raw	3½ oz	100

Meat: Pork

bacon

Canadian, grilled	2 slices	85
cured		
raw	2 slices	250
pan fried, broiled	2 slices	75
thick sliced, pan fried, broiled	2 slices	120

belly (see *Organ Meats*)

bologna (see *Luncheon and Deli Meats*)

brain (see *Organ Meats*)

bratwurst (see *Luncheon and Deli Meats*)

Food	Serving Size	Calories

Meat: Pork *(continued)*

braunschweiger (see *Luncheon and Deli Meats*)

brotwurst (see *Luncheon and Deli Meats*)

chitterlings (see *Organ Meats*)

chorizo (see *Luncheon and Deli Meats*)

ear (see *Organ Meats*)

feet (see *Organ Meats*)

frankfurter (see *Luncheon and Deli Meats*)

ham (cured)		
roasted	3½ oz	180
canned	3½ oz	190
loaf (see *Luncheon and Deli Meats*)		
patty	2½ oz patty	205
steak	3½ oz	120

headcheese (see *Luncheon and Deli Meats*)

heart (see *Organ Meats*)

hot dog (see *Luncheon and Deli Meats: frankfurter*)

jowl (see *Organ Meats*)

kidney (see *Organ Meats*)

Food	Serving Size	Calories

Meat: Pork *(continued)*

kielbasa (see *Luncheon and Deli Meats*)

knockwurst (see *Luncheon and Deli Meats*)

leg

roasted, lean and fat	3½ oz	275
roasted, lean	3½ oz	210

liver (see *Organ Meats*)

liverwurst (see *Luncheon and Deli Meats*)

loin

braised, lean and fat	3½ oz	240
braised, lean	3½ oz	205
broiled, lean and fat	3½ oz	240
broiled, lean	3½ oz	210
roasted, lean and fat	3½ oz	250
roasted, lean	3½ oz	210

loin blade (chop, roast)

braised, lean and fat	3½ oz	325
braised, lean	3½ oz	225
broiled, lean and fat	3½ oz	320
broiled, lean	3½ oz	235
pan fried, lean and fat	3½ oz	240
pan fried, lean	3½ oz	240
roasted, lean and fat	3½ oz	325
roasted, lean	3½ oz	245

lung (see *Organ Meats*)

Food	Serving Size	Calories

Meat: Pork *(continued)*

pancreas (see *Organ Meats*)

picnic
cured, roasted, lean and fat	3½ oz	280
cured, roasted, lean	3½ oz	170
braised, lean and fat	3½ oz	330
braised, lean	3½ oz	250
roasted, lean and fat	3½ oz	315
roasted, lean	3½ oz	230

pepperoni (see *Luncheon and Deli Meats*)

rib (chop, roast)
braised, lean and fat	3½ oz	255
braised, lean	3½ oz	210
broiled, lean and fat	3½ oz	260
broiled, lean	3½ oz	215
pan fried, lean and fat	3½ oz	225
pan fried, lean	3½ oz	225
roasted, lean and fat	3½ oz	250
roasted, lean	3½ oz	215
sparerib, braised	3½ oz	295

rolled roast | 3½ oz | 285

rump
roasted, lean and fat	3½ oz	250
roasted, lean	3½ oz	205

salami (see *Luncheon and Deli Meats*)

Meat and Poultry

Food	Serving Size	Calories
Meat: Pork *(continued)*		
sausage		
breakfast link, patty	1 oz	100
italian	2½ oz	215
shank		
roasted, lean and fat	3½ oz	290
roasted, lean	3½ oz	215
shoulder		
roasted, lean and fat	3½ oz	290
roasted, lean	3½ oz	230
spleen (see *Organ Meats*)		
stomach (see *Organ Meats*)		
tail (see *Organ Meats*)		
tenderloin		
roasted, lean and fat	3½ oz	175
roasted, lean	3½ oz	165
tongue (see *Organ Meats*)		
Meat: Veal		
brain, calf (see *Organ Meats*)		
bockwurst (see *Luncheon and Deli Meats*)		
cubes	3½ oz	190

Food	Serving Size	Calories

Meat: Veal *(continued)*

ground, broiled 3½ oz 170

heart (see *Organ Meats*)

kidney (see *Organ Meats*)

leg
cutlet, pan fried

breaded	3½ oz	230
not breaded	3½ oz	210

liver, calf (see *Organ Meats*)

loin

braised, lean and fat	3½ oz	285
braised, lean	3½ oz	225
roasted, lean and fat	3½ oz	215
roasted, lean	3½ oz	175

lung (see *Organ Meats*)

pancreas (see *Organ Meats*)

rib

braised, lean and fat	3½ oz	250
braised, lean	3½ oz	220
roasted, lean and fat	3½ oz	230
roasted, lean	3½ oz	175

shoulder

braised, lean and fat	3½ oz	235

Food	Serving Size	Calories

Meat: Veal *(continued)*

shoulder *(continued)*

braised, lean	3½ oz	200
roasted, lean and fat	3½ oz	185
roasted, lean	3½ oz	165

sirloin

braised, lean and fat	3½ oz	250
braised, lean	3½ oz	205
roasted, lean and fat	3½ oz	200
roasted, lean	3½ oz	170

spleen (see *Organ Meats*)

sweetbreads (see *Organ Meats*)

tongue (see *Organ Meats*)

Poultry: Chicken

prepared slices, salad (see *Luncheon and Deli Meats*)

whole, broiler/fryer

dark meat, with skin

roasted	3½ oz	255
stewed	3½ oz	235

dark meat, without skin

roasted	3½ oz	205
stewed	3½ oz	190

light meat, with skin

roasted	3½ oz	220
stewed	3½ oz	200

Food	Serving Size	Calories
Poultry: Chicken *(continued)*		
whole, broiler/fryer *(continued)*		
light meat, without skin		
roasted	3½ oz	175
stewed	3½ oz	160
light and dark meat, with skin		
roasted	3½ oz	240
stewed	3½ oz	220
light and dark meat, without skin		
roasted	3½ oz	190
stewed	3½ oz	175
whole, capon, with skin, roasted	3½ oz	230
whole, roaster		
dark meat, without skin, roasted	3½ oz	180
light meat, without skin, roasted	3½ oz	155
dark/light meat, with skin, roasted	3½ oz	225
whole, stewer		
dark meat, without skin, stewed	3½ oz	260
light meat without skin, stewed	3½ oz	215
light/dark meat, with skin, stewed	3½ oz	285
parts		
back, with skin, fried	2½ oz	240
breast, with skin		
fried, flour coated	½ breast	220
fried, battered	½ breast	370
roasted	½ breast	195
stewed	½ breast	200

Food	Serving Size	Calories

Poultry: Chicken (continued)

parts (continued)

breast, without skin

fried, flour coated	½ breast	160
roasted	½ breast	140
stewed	½ breast	145
cutlet (skinless, boneless), raw	4 oz	130

drumstick, with skin (lower leg only)

fried, flour coated	1; approx 1¾ oz	120
fried, battered	1; approx 2½ oz	195
roasted	1; approx 1¾ oz	110
stewed	1; approx 1¾ oz	115

leg, with skin (drumstick and thigh)

fried, flour coated	1; approx 4 oz	285
roasted	1; approx 4 oz	265
stewed	1; approx 4 oz	275

neck, simmered

with skin	1 neck	95
without skin	1 neck	30

thigh, with skin

fried, flour coated	1; approx 2 oz	160
fried, battered	1; approx 3 oz	240
roasted	1; approx 2 oz	155
stewed	1; approx 2 oz	160

thigh, without skin

roasted	1; approx 2 oz	110

wing, with skin

fried, flour coated	1; approx 1 oz	105
fried, battered	1; approx 1½ oz	160
roasted	1; approx 1 oz	100
stewed	1; approx 1 oz	100
spicy*	3; approx 3 oz	170

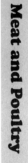

Meat and Poultry

Food	Serving Size	Calories

Poultry: Chicken *(continued)*

nuggets, breaded*	6 pieces; approx 3 oz	275
patty*	1 patty; approx 2½ oz	185

Poultry: Organs

gizzard
chicken, simmered	3½ oz	155
goose, raw	3½ oz	140
turkey, simmered	3½ oz	165

heart
chicken, simmered	3½ oz	185
turkey, simmered	3½ oz	175

liver
chicken, simmered	3½ oz	155
duck, raw	3½ oz	135
goose, raw	3½ oz	150
turkey, simmered	3½ oz	170

Poultry: Turkey

prepared breast (see *Luncheon and Deli Meats*)

whole, roasted
dark meat, with skin	3½ oz	220
dark meat, without skin	3½ oz	185

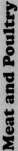

*Average calories; calorie counts vary widely among brands and recipes.

Food	Serving Size	Calories
Poultry: Turkey *(continued)*		
whole, roasted *(continued)*		
light meat, with skin	3½ oz	195
light meat, without skin	3½ oz	155
ground, raw	4 oz	175
nuggets, breaded*	4 pieces; approx 3¼ oz	255
patty, breaded, uncooked*	3 oz	215
Poultry: Other		
cornish game hen		
roasted, with skin	½ bird; approx 4 oz	295
roasted, without skin	½ bird; approx 4 oz	145
duck		
roasted, with skin	3½ oz	335
roasted, without skin	3½ oz	200
goose		
roasted, with skin	3½ oz	305
roasted, without skin	3½ oz	240
pheasant, with skin, raw	3½ oz	180
quail, without skin, raw	3½ oz	135

*Average calories; calorie counts vary widely among brands and recipes.

Food	Serving Size	Calories
Luncheon and Deli Meats*		
beef loaf (lunch meat)	2 oz	86
blood sausage (blood pudding)	1 oz	95
bockwurst, uncooked	1 link	200
bologna		
beef	1 oz	90
light (reduced fat)	1 oz	55
beef and pork	1 oz	90
chicken, pork, and beef	1 oz	90
lebanon	1 oz	60
pork	1 oz	70
turkey	1 oz	56
turkey, beef, and pork, fat free	1 oz	23
bratwurst	3 oz link	255
braunschweiger	1 oz	95
brotwurst	2½ oz link	225
chicken roll	1 oz	50
chorizo	2 oz link	275
corned beef	2 oz	120

*Average calories; calorie counts vary widely among brands.

Food	Serving Size	Calories
Luncheon and Deli Meats (continued)		
frankfurter		
beef	2 oz link; 8/lb	180
fat free	2 oz link; 8/lb	54
beef and pork	2 oz link; 8/lb	180
chicken	1½ oz link; 10/lb	115
pork and turkey	1½ oz link; 10/lb	145
pork, turkey, and beef, light	2 oz link; 8/lb	110
turkey	1½ oz link; 10/lb	100
turkey and beef, fat free	1¾ oz link	35
turkey and chicken	1½ oz link; 10/lb	80
turkey, chicken, and beef, fat free	2 oz link; 8/lb	55
ham and cheese		
loaf	1 oz	65
spread	1 oz	70
ham, deli style (also see *Meat: Pork*)		
baked	2 oz	60
boiled	2 oz	60
deviled	⅓ cup; 3 oz	210
glazed	2 oz	60
minced, loaf	2 oz	145
salad spread	1 oz	60
smoked	2 oz	55
turkey	2 oz	75
headcheese	1 oz	60
hot dog (see *frankfurter*)		
kielbasa	1 oz	85

Food	Serving Size	Calories
Luncheon and Deli Meats *(continued)*		
knockwurst	1 oz	85
liver pâté		
chicken	1 oz	55
goose (foie gras)	1 oz	130
liverwurst	1 oz	90
mortadella	2 oz	175
olive loaf	1 oz	65
pastrami		
beef	1 oz	40
turkey	1 oz	40
pepperoni	1 oz	140
pimento loaf	1 oz	75
salami		
beef	1 oz	75
beef and pork	1 oz	60
cooked (cotto)		
beef, chicken, and pork	1 oz	70
beef	1 oz	55
turkey	1 oz	45
dry/hard		
pork	1 oz	115
pork and beef	1 oz	115
genoa	1 oz	105
turkey	1 oz	40

Food	Serving Size	Calories

Luncheon and Deli Meats (continued)

smoked link sausage

beef	1½ oz link	130
pork	2½ oz link	265
pork and beef	2½ oz link	230
pork and turkey	2 oz link	170

thuringer

beef and pork	1 oz	80
beef	1 oz	85

turkey breast
roasted

fat free	2 oz	50
with skin	3½ oz	125
smoked	1 oz	30
fat free	2 oz	50

turkey ham (see *ham*)

turkey pastrami (see *pastrami*)

turkey salami (see *salami*)

Vienna sausage
reduced fat

25%	1.9 oz; 3 links	130
50%	1.9 oz; 3 links	90
beef and pork	1¾ oz; 3 links	135
chicken	1¾ oz; 3 links	100
in barbecue sauce	2 oz; 3 links, sauce	140
smoked	2 oz; 3 links	150

Food	Serving Size	Calories

Meat and Poultry Substitutes*

bacon

strips	½ oz; 2 strips	50
bits	1½ tbsp	30

bean/lentil loaf	3 oz	150

breakfast sausage

links	1 oz; 1 link	65
patty	1⅓ oz; 1 patty	95

burger	2 oz	60

"chicken"

nuggets	3 oz; 5 pieces	245
patty	2½ oz	175

frankfurter	2 oz; 1 piece	100

meat extender	1 oz	90

*Average calories; calorie counts vary widely among brands.

Food	Serving Size	Calories

Nuts*

almonds
whole	1 oz	165
chopped	1 oz	175
sliced, slivered	1 oz	170
dry roasted	1 oz	165
oil roasted	1 oz	175
honey roasted	1 oz	170
barbecue flavor	1 oz	165
meal	1 oz	115
butter	1 tbsp	100
paste	1 oz	130

brazil nuts	1 oz	185

cashews
dry roasted	1 oz	165
oil roasted	1 oz	165
honey roasted	1 oz	150
butter	1 oz	165

chestnuts, fresh, roasted	1 oz	70
water chestnuts (see *Vegetables*)		

coconut
fresh	1 oz	100
dried, shredded		
sweetened	1 cup	465
unsweetened	1 oz	185
cream, sweetened	1 cup	570

*Edible portion only (no shells), unless otherwise indicated.

Food	Serving Size	Calories

Nuts (continued)

coconut (continued)

milk	1 cup	550
water	1 cup	46

filberts (see *hazelnuts*)

hazelnuts

whole	1 oz	165
chopped, sliced	1 oz	160
dry roasted	1 oz	190
oil roasted	1 oz	190
butter	1 tbsp	100
with chocolate (Nutella)	1 tbsp	80
hickory	1 oz	185

macadamia

dry roasted	1 oz	200
oil roasted	1 oz	205

mixed

dry roasted	1 oz	170
honey roasted	1 oz	170
oil roasted	1 oz	175

peanuts

raw	1 oz	160
dry roasted	1 oz	165
honey roasted	1 oz	150
roasted in oil	1 oz	165

Nuts and Seeds

Food	Serving Size	Calories
Nuts (continued)		
peanuts (continued)		
Spanish		
raw	1 oz	160
oil roasted	1 oz	165
peanut butter*		
creamy, smooth	2 tbsp	190
chunky	2 tbsp	188
reduced fat	2 tbsp	190
with jelly	2 tbsp	180
pecans		
halves	1 oz	190
chopped	½ cup	380
oil roasted	1 oz	195
honey roasted	1 oz	200
pine nuts (pignoli)	1 oz	160
pistachios		
in shells	2 oz	165
shelled	1 oz	165
soy nuts		
dry roasted	1 oz	125
oil roasted	1 oz	130
walnuts		
whole, halves	1 oz	190

*Average calories; calorie counts vary widely among brands.

Nuts and Seeds

127

Food	Serving Size	Calories

Nuts *(continued)*

walnuts *(continued)*

chopped	1 cup	760
ground	½ cup	240

Seeds*

flax	1 oz	140
pumpkin	1 oz	155

sesame

raw	1 tbsp	45
toasted	1 oz	160
tahini (sesame paste)		
raw	1 tbsp	85
toasted	1 tbsp	90

sunflower

raw	1 oz	160
toasted	1 oz	175
dry roasted	1 oz	165
oil roasted	1 oz	175

Nuts and Seeds

*See *Extras: Herbs and Spices* for herb and spice seeds.

Food	Serving Size	Calories
Chips and Nibbles*		
banana chips	1 oz	140
beef stick, smoked	½ oz stick	50
beef jerky	.7 oz piece	80
Bugles	1½ cup	160
carrot chips	1 oz	60
cheese balls, curls	1 oz	150
reduced fat	1 oz	130
cheese puffs	1 oz	155
cheese straws	5 pieces; approx 1 oz	135
Chex mix	1 oz	130
corn chips		
plain	1 oz	155
nacho	1 oz	145
tortilla	1 oz	140

Cracker Jack (see *popcorn, caramel coated*)

Snack Foods

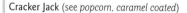

*Except for brand name items, average calories; calorie counts vary widely among brands. Read the label and pay attention to serving size as pack-aged sizes vary widely.

Food	Serving Size	Calories

Chips and Nibbles *(continued)*

crackers (also see *Breads, Crackers, and Baked Goods*)

Food	Serving Size	Calories
Goldfish	1 oz	140
mix, snack, party	1 oz	160
oriental	1 oz	155
popcorn		
kernels, unpopped	¼ cup	180
air popped (no fat added)	1 oz; approx 3½ cups	20
oil popped	1 oz; approx 3½ cups	55
microwave		
buttered	1 oz; approx 3½ cups	35
light	1 oz; approx 3½ cups	25
bagged	1 oz; approx 3½ cups	160
movie theater		
small	approx 7 cups	400
buttered	approx 7 cups	580
medium	approx 16 cups	900
buttered	approx 16 cups	1170
large	approx 20 cups	1150
buttered	approx 20 cups	1500
caramel coated	1 oz	120
pork rinds	1 oz	155
potato chips		
plain	1 oz	150
reduced fat	1 oz	135
no fat (made with Olestra)	1 oz	75
flavored (barbecue, onion, garlic, sour cream and onion, etc.)	1 oz	140

Snack Foods

Food	Serving Size	Calories
Chips and Nibbles (continued)		
potato chips (continued)		
cheese	1 oz	140
sweet potato	1 oz	150
potato sticks	1 oz	140
pretzels		
regular	1 oz	110
chocolate coated	1 oz	130
soft	2½ oz	190
rice cakes (see *Breads, Crackers, and Baked Goods*)		
vegetable chips	1 oz	130
Dips and Spreads		
avocado (guacamole)	2 tbsp	60
baba gannouj (eggplant/tahini)	2 tbsp	70
bean	2 tbsp	40
blue cheese	2 tbsp	80
cheese	2 tbsp	90
clam	2 tbsp	50
hummus (chickpeas/tahini)	2 tbsp	50

Food	Serving Size	Calories
Dips and Spreads *(continued)*		
jalapeño	2 tbsp	30
nacho	2 tbsp	60
pâté (also see *Meat and Poultry: Luncheon and Deli Meats*)		
smoked salmon	1 oz	45
spinach	1 oz	50
salsa	2 tbsp	10
sour cream–onion		
regular	2 tbsp	50
low fat	2 tbsp	40
sour cream–onion–bacon, regular	2 tbsp	60
spinach	2 tbsp	70
taramasalata (fish roe)		
regular	1 tbsp	90
light	1 tbsp	40
vegetable	2 tbsp	30
low fat	2 tbsp	25
yogurt-cucumber (tzatziki)	2 tbsp	40
Energy Bars		
breakfast	1⅓ oz bar	130
granola	1⅓ oz bar	135

Food	Serving Size	Calories

Energy Bars *(continued)*

fruit	1⅓ oz bar	125
low fat	1 oz bar	110
peanut butter	1 oz bar	120

Sweet Snacks: Candy

bars

Almond Joy	1.7 oz bar	240
Baby Ruth	2.1 oz bar	290
Bit-O-Honey	1.7 oz bar	185
Butterfinger	2.16 oz bar	295
Charleston Chew	1.9 oz bar	230
Fifth Avenue	2 oz bar	195
Heath	1.4 oz bar	210
Kit Kat	1.5 oz bar	220
Mars	1.8 oz bar	235
Milky Way	2.15 oz bar	260
Mounds	1.9 oz bar	255
Mr. Goodbar	1¾ oz bar	250
Nestlé Crunch	1.4 oz bar	210
Oh Henry!	2 oz bar	245
Snickers	2.16 oz bar	290
Three Musketeers	2.13 oz bar	250

bits

after dinner mints	1 piece	15
butterscotch	1 oz	110
candy corn	1 oz	110
caramel	2½ oz	270
chocolate-covered (see *chocolate*)		
Good & Plenty	1 oz	105

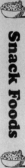

Snack Foods

Food	Serving Size	Calories

Sweet Snacks: Candy *(continued)*

bits *(continued)*

Good & Fruity	1 oz	75
gumdrops	1 oz	110
gummies	1⅓ oz	130
hard candy (sour balls)	1 oz	105
sugar free	1 oz	80
Jelly Beans	1 oz	105
Jordan almonds (candy coated)	1 oz	130
Life Savers	1 piece	10
licorice (see *Sweet Snacks: Candy: licorice*)		
M&Ms		
regular	1.69 oz bag	235
peanut	1.74 oz bag	255
malted milk balls	1⅓ oz	160
maple sugar candy	1 oz	100
mint lozenges	1 oz	100
Necco wafers	2 oz	15
nougat	1 oz	115
Now and Later	1 pkg	270
Peppermint Patties	1½ oz	165
Reese's Peanut Butter Cups	1.8 oz	280
Reese's Pieces	1.6 oz	225
saltwater taffy	1 oz	110
spearmint leaves (see *gumdrops*)		
Skittles	2⅓ oz	265
Starburst	2.07 oz	235
Tic Tac	1 piece	1.5
toffee	½ oz	70
Tootsie Rolls	1 piece	25

bubble gum (see *gum*)

Food	Serving Size	Calories

Sweet Snacks: Candy *(continued)*

candy cane	½ oz	50
carob		
bar	1 oz	155
carob-coated nuts	1 oz	150
carob-coated raisins	1 oz	125
chewing gum (see *gum*)		
chocolate		
baking (see *Sweets and Desserts: Baking Ingredients*)		
dark	1 oz	150
with nuts	1 oz	160
milk	1 oz	150
with nuts	1 oz	160
fudge	1 oz	110
with nuts	1 oz	120
chocolate coffee beans	1 oz	130
chocolate-covered cherry	1	55
chocolate-covered mints	1 oz	115
chocolate-covered nuts	1 oz	160
chocolate-covered raisins	1 oz	120
with filled centers	1 oz	125
Hershey's Kisses	1 oz	200
truffles	½ oz	55
cough drops	1 drop	15
fruit leather/rolls	1 oz	95

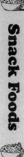

Snack Foods

Food	Serving Size	Calories

Sweet Snacks: Candy *(continued)*

fruit peel (see *Fruits: citrus peel*)

Food	Serving Size	Calories
gum		
bubble	1 stick	25
sugar free	1 stick	15
chewing	1 stick	10
sugar free	1 stick	5
halvah	1 oz	185
licorice		
bits	1 oz	10
twists	1 piece	30
laces	1 piece	35
lollipops		
small	1	20
medium	1	30
large	1	40
Tootsie Pop	1	50
marshmallow		
regular	1 piece	25
miniature	1 cup	145
fluff	2 tbsp	40
marzipan	1 oz	140
peanut brittle	1 oz	130

Food	Serving Size	Calories
Sweet Snacks: Candy *(continued)*		
praline	1 oz	130
sesame bar	1 oz	145
trail mix	2 oz	250
yogurt-covered raisins	1 oz	120

Snack Foods

Food	Serving Size	Calories

Note: For home recipes, use values for individual ingredients to determine total calories.

Soups*

asparagus, cream of
canned, reconstituted
made with milk	I cup	160
made with water	I cup	85
made from mix	I cup	60

bean
black, canned, reconstituted	I cup	115
with bacon		
canned, reconstituted	I cup	170
made from mix	I cup	105
with franks, canned, reconstituted	I cup	190

beef
bouillon, cube or powder	I cube or I tsp	5
broth	I cup	20
consommé	I cup	50
tomato beef noodle	I cup	140
with mushrooms	I cup	75
with noodles		
canned, reconstituted	I cup	85
made from mix	I cup	40

*Average calories; calorie counts vary widely among brands. Calorie counts are based on a I-cup serving; many containers hold more than one serving, so read the label.

Food	Serving Size	Calories
Soups *(continued)*		
beef *(continued)*		
with vegetables, canned	1 cup	135
fat free	1 cup	135
and barley, canned, reconstituted	1 cup	80
borscht	1 cup	105
low calorie	1 cup	25
broccoli		
cream of		
canned, reconstituted	1 cup	100
fat free	1 cup	80
with cheese	1 cup	110
fat free	1 cup	80
cauliflower, made from mix	1 cup	70
celery, cream of		
canned, reconstituted		
made with milk	1 cup	165
made with water	1 cup	90
made from mix	1 cup	65
cheese		
canned, reconstituted		
made with milk	1 cup	230
made with water	1 cup	155
chicken		
bouillon, cube or powder	1 cube or 1 tsp	5

Food	Serving Size	Calories
Soups (continued)		
chicken (continued)		
broth	I cup	40
fat free	I cup	30
cream of, canned, reconstituted		
made with milk	I cup	190
made with water	I cup	115
made from mix	I cup	105
gumbo, canned, reconstituted	I cup	55
with dumplings, canned,		
reconstituted	I cup	95
with matzo balls, home recipe	I cup	180
with noodles		
canned, reconstituted	I cup	75
fat free	I cup	75
made from mix	I cup	55
with rice		
canned, reconstituted	I cup	60
made from mix	I cup	60
with vegetables		
canned, reconstituted	I cup	75
made from mix	I cup	50
clam chowder		
Manhattan style		
canned, reconstituted	I cup	80
made from mix	I cup	65
New England style		
canned, reconstituted		
made with milk	I cup	165
made with water	I cup	95
made from mix	I cup	95

Food	Serving Size	Calories
Soups *(continued)*		
French onion (see *onion*)		
gazpacho	1 cup	55
leek, made from mix	1 cup	70
lentil		
canned, reconstituted	1 cup	130
fat free	1 cup	110
made from mix	1 cup	130
minestrone		
canned, reconstituted	1 cup	80
fat free	1 cup	110
made from mix	1 cup	80
mushroom		
canned, reconstituted	1 cup	85
made from mix	1 cup	95
cream of		
canned, reconstituted		
made with milk	1 cup	205
made with water	1 cup	130
made from mix	6 oz	60
with barley	1 cup	75
onion		
canned, reconstituted	1 cup	60
cream of		
made with milk	1 cup	185
made with water	1 cup	110

Food	Serving Size	Calories
Soups *(continued)*		
onion *(continued)*		
made from mix	1 cup	25
oyster stew, canned, reconstituted		
made with milk	1 cup	135
made with water	1 cup	60
pasta e fagioli, home recipe	1 cup	195
pea, split		
canned, reconstituted		
made with milk	1 cup	240
made with water	1 cup	165
with ham, made with water	1 cup	190
made from mix	1 cup	135
pepperpot, canned, reconstituted	1 cup	100
potato, cream of		
canned, reconstituted		
made with milk	1 cup	150
made with water	1 cup	75
ramen noodle		
beef	2 oz pkg	290
chicken	2 oz pkg	290
pork	1½ oz pkg	170
shrimp	1½ oz pkg	170
Scotch broth, canned, reconstituted	1 cup	80

Food	Serving Size	Calories
Soups *(continued)*		
shrimp, cream of		
canned, reconstituted		
made with milk	I cup	165
made with water	I cup	90
tomato, canned, reconstituted		
made with milk	I cup	160
made with water	I cup	85
made from mix	I cup	105
bisque		
made with milk	I cup	200
made with water	I cup	125
with rice	I cup	120
with vegetables	I cup	80
turkey		
with noodles	I cup	70
with vegetables	I cup	70
vegetable		
bouillon, cube or powder	I cube or I tsp	5
broth	I cup	15
with beef, canned, reconstituted	I cup	80
fat free	I cup	70
vegetarian	I cup	70
vichyssoise (see *potato, cream of*)		
wonton	I cup	180

Food	Serving Size	Calories

Packaged Entrées*

Hamburger Helper (as prepared, with ground beef)

Food	Serving Size	Calories
Beef Romanoff	l cup	290
Beef Stew	l cup	250
Beef Teriyaki	l cup	290
Cheddar Melt	l cup	310
Cheddar Primavera	l cup	320
Cheeseburger Macaroni	l cup	360
Cheesy Italian	l cup	330
Chili Macaroni	l cup	290
Fettucini Alfredo	l cup	310
Hamburger Stew	l cup	250
Italian Rigatoni	l cup	180
Lasagna	l cup	280
Meat Loaf	l cup	280
Mushrooms and Wild Rice	l cup	310
Nacho Cheese	l cup	320
Pizzabake	l cup	270
Potatoes au Gratin	l cup	290
Rice Oriental	l cup	310
Salisbury	l cup	270
Stroganoff	l cup	320
Swedish Meatball	l cup	300
Zesty Italian	l cup	320
Zesty Mexican	l cup	300

*No attempt has been made to include all packaged and frozen entrées since full nutritional information is available on the label. Except for brand name items, average calories; calorie counts vary widely among brands and recipes. Calorie counts are based on a l-cup serving; many containers hold more than one serving.

Food	Serving Size	Calories

Packaged Entrées (continued)

Pizza (frozen)

cheese	3½ oz	250
combination	3½ oz	265
pepperoni	3½ oz	260
sausage	3½ oz	255
French bread style		
cheese	5¾ oz	390
pepperoni	6 oz	425
sausage	6¼ oz	405
Lean Cuisine		
cheese	5 oz	310
pepperoni	5½ oz	340
sausage	6 oz	330

Pot Pie

beef	1 pie; approx 7 oz	350
chicken	1 pie; approx 7 oz	365
turkey	1 pie; approx 7 oz	375
vegetable and cheese	1 pie; approx 7 oz	390

Tuna Helper (as prepared with canned tuna)

Au Gratin	1 cup	310
Cheesy Pasta	1 cup	280
Creamy Broccoli	1 cup	310
Creamy Pasta	1 cup	300
Fettucine Alfredo	1 cup	310
Garden Cheddar	1 cup	310
Pasta Salad	¾ cup	380
Tetrazzini	1 cup	310
Tuna Romanoff	1 cup	280

Food	Serving Size	Calories
Mexican Specialties		
burrito		
bean and cheese	1; approx 3 oz	190
beef	1; approx 4 oz	265
chicken	1; approx 4 oz	260
chili		
beans only	1 cup	240
con carne	1 cup	285
meat only	1 cup	370
enchilada		
beef	5.7 oz	200
cheese	5.7 oz	170
fajita (fast food style)		
chicken	1; approx 8 oz	460
steak	1; approx 8 oz	465
menudo	1 cup	110
nachos	approx 3½ oz	325
quesadilla	1	370
taco	1; approx 6 oz	370
tamale	2; approx 6 oz	270
tostada (beef, beans, cheese)	1; approx 8 oz	335

Food	Serving Size	Calories
Noodle Dishes		
beef and noodles	1 cup	300
beef stroganoff	1 cup	440
chicken and noodles	1 cup	365
chow mein	1 cup	255
noodles romanoff	3 oz	130
tuna noodle casserole	6 oz	195
turkey tetrazzini	6 oz	240
Pasta Dishes		
pasta (all shapes)		
with broccoli and cheese	1 cup	390
with cheddar	1 cup	280
with three cheese	1 cup	320
with four cheese	1 cup	290
with marinara sauce	8 oz	240
with meatballs	1 cup	330
with meat sauce	1 cup	375
primavera	8 oz	250
with oil and garlic	1 cup	325
with pesto sauce	1 cup	350
with sausage and tomato sauce	8 oz	350
with tomato sauce	1 cup	260
salad	8 oz	220

Food	Serving Size	Calories
Pasta Dishes (continued)		
cannelloni	6 oz	280
fettucine Alfredo	8 oz	350
gnocchi, with tomato sauce	8 oz	300
lasagna with meat and tomato sauce	8 oz	360
macaroni and cheese	1 cup	320
manicotti with cheese and tomato sauce	8 oz	230
ravioli, beef with sauce	8 oz	300
tortellini, cheese with tomato sauce	5½ oz	260
Rice Dishes		
fried rice (Chinese)	1 cup	235
pilaf	½ cup	115
risotto	1 cup	420
Spanish rice	½ cup	195
white and wild rice pilaf	½ cup	240

Food	Serving Size	Calories
Rice Dishes (continued)		
yellow rice (Mexican)	½ cup	160
Stews		
beef and vegetable	1 cup	195
beef burgundy	7½ oz	315
bouillabaise	1 cup	200
Brunswick stew	1 cup	230
chicken à la king	1 cup	470
chicken and dumplings	7 oz	290
chicken cacciatore	7 oz	280
chicken fricassee	1 cup	385
chipped beef, creamed	1 cup	375
moussaka	8 oz	350
osso buco (excluding bones)	8 oz	550
oyster stew	1 cup	235
pot roast, beef	7½ oz	250

Food	Serving Size	Calories
Miscellaneous		
cheese fondue	½ cup	250
corned beef hash	1 cup	440
crab cake	1 piece; approx 2 oz	95
croquettes		
chicken, with gravy	2 pieces; approx 5¾ oz	340
ham	1 piece; approx 2½ oz	165
dolma (stuffed grape leaves)	3 pieces	200
egg roll (chinese)	1 piece; approx 3 oz	170
escargots (snails), garlic butter	6	200
falafel	3 pieces; approx 3 oz	175
fish loaf	1 slice; approx 5 oz	180
fish patty	1 piece; approx 3 oz	200
fritters		
clam	1 piece; approx 1¼ oz	125
corn	1 piece; approx 1 oz	130
frog legs (raw, meat only)	4 oz	85
meat loaf	1 slice; approx 3 oz	155

Food	Serving Size	Calories

Miscellaneous *(continued)*

quiche
Lorraine	1 piece; approx 3 oz	400
spinach and mushroom	1 piece; approx 3 oz	240

soufflé
cheese	1 cup	205
spinach	1 cup	220

spanakopita	3 oz	350
stuffed cabbage (with beef and rice)	1 piece; approx 7 oz	200
stuffed pepper (with beef and rice)	1 piece; approx 6½ oz	315
veal marsala	8 oz	300
veal parmigiana	8 oz	350
Welsh rarebit	1 cup	415

Food	Serving Size	Calories
Baking Ingredients		
baking powder	I tsp	5
baking soda	I tsp	0
Bisquick		
regular	I cup	510
reduced fat	I cup	450
chocolate		
unsweetened	I oz	150
semisweet	I oz	160
white	I oz	160
chips		
semisweet	I oz	140
mint	I oz	150
peanut butter	I oz	160
white	I oz	80
cocoa powder	I tbsp	10
cornstarch	I tbsp	30
cream of tartar	I tsp	10
flour (also see *Cereals, Grains, Pasta, and Rice*)		
arrowroot	I cup	445
buckwheat	I cup	400
carob	I cup	185
corn	I cup	415
potato	I cup	630
rice, brown	I cup	575

Food	Serving Size	Calories
Baking Ingredients (continued)		
flour (also see *Cereals, Grains, Pasta, and Rice*) (continued)		
rice, white	1 cup	600
rye, dark	1 cup	415
rye, medium	1 cup	360
rye, light	1 cup	375
self-rising	1 cup	445
semolina	1 cup	600
soy	1 cup	370
low fat	1 cup	285
white	1 cup	455
whole wheat	1 cup	405
graham cracker crumbs	1 cup	360
pie crust (see *Pies, Fillings, and Crusts*)		
yeast	¼ oz pkg	20
Cakes*		
angel food	1 oz; ¹⁄₁₂ cake	75
apple crumb	2 oz	260
banana, frosted	2½ oz	370
black forest	1½ oz	350

Sweets and Desserts

*Average calories; calorie counts vary widely among brands and recipes. Unless otherwise noted, cakes are without icing; for iced cake, add calorie value of 2 tbsp/1 oz icing per serving.

Food	Serving Size	Calories
Cakes *(continued)*		
brownie	1 piece; 2 oz	225
with nuts	1 piece; 2 oz	240
bundt	3 oz slice	300
carrot		
plain	2½ oz slice	240
with cream cheese icing	2½ oz slice	380
cheese		
plain	2¾ oz slice	255
with fruit topping	5 oz slice	410
low fat	3 oz slice	150
chocolate		
plain	3½ oz slice	340
with frosting	4 oz slice	375
pudding-style	2¾ oz slice	270
fat free	1½ oz slice	170
cinnamon crumb	4 oz slice	450
coconut, with icing	3 oz slice	360
coffee	2 oz slice	265
cupcake		
with chocolate icing	1¾ oz	175
with white icing	1¾ oz	170

Sweets and Desserts

Food	Serving Size	Calories

Cakes *(continued)*

devil's food

plain	1½ oz slice	190
with chocolate icing	3 oz slice	325
reduced fat	1½ oz slice	220
fruit	1½ oz piece	140
gingerbread	2½ oz piece	265

lemon

	2¾ oz slice	250
chiffon	2 oz slice	140
fat free	1½ oz slice	170
pudding-style	3 oz slice	180
with poppy seeds	3 oz slice	210
marble	2½ oz slice	250
pineapple upside down	4 oz piece	365
pound	2 oz slice	230

snack cakes

Devil Dog	1½ oz	170
Ding Dong	1 piece; approx 1½ oz	180
Drake's coffee cake	1 oz	130
Ho-Ho	1 piece; 1 oz	125
Ring-Ding	1 piece; approx 1½ oz	165
Sno Ball	1; approx 1¾ oz	180
Tastykake low fat lemon cupcake	1 piece; 1 oz	80
Twinkies	2 pieces; 1½ oz	150
light	2 pieces; 1½ oz	140

Sweets and Desserts

Food	Serving Size	Calories
Cakes *(continued)*		
snack cakes *(continued)*		
Yodels	I piece; approx I oz	280
spice	3 oz slice	250
sponge	2 oz slice	185
tiramisu	4 oz piece	320
white	2½ oz slice	265
with coconut icing	4 oz slice	400
reduced fat	1½ oz slice	210
yellow	2½ oz slice	245
with chocolate icing	3½ oz slice	380
with white icing	3½ oz slice	375
light	I oz slice	115
pudding-style	2½ oz slice	245

Cake Frostings, Icings, and Fillings*

Food	Serving Size	Calories
butter cream	2 tbsp	150
butterscotch	2 tbsp	140
caramel	2 tbsp	140
cake and cookie decoration		
chocolate	I tbsp	65
all other flavors	I tbsp	76

*Average calories; calorie counts vary widely among brands and recipes.

Food	Serving Size	Calories
Cake Frostings, Icings, and Fillings *(continued)*		
chocolate		
home recipe, creamy	2 tbsp	100
home recipe, glaze	2 tbsp	95
ready made, creamy	2 tbsp	110
low fat	2 tbsp	120
cream filling (boiled)	½ cup	165
cream cheese	2 tbsp	155
fudge	2 tbsp	140
lemon	2 tbsp	140
mocha, ready made	2 tbsp	130
sour cream	2 tbsp	155
sugar icing/glaze, home recipe	2 tbsp	100
vanilla		
home recipe	2 tbsp	165
ready made	2 tbsp	140
light	2 tbsp	120
white, boiled, home recipe	2 tbsp	100
Candy (see *Snack Foods: Sweet Snacks*)		

Sweets and Desserts

Food	Serving Size	Calories
Cookies*		
almond	1 oz	140
anisette	1 oz	90
biscotti	1 oz	100
butter	1 oz	130
chocolate	1 oz	140
mint	1 oz	150
chocolate chip		
small	½ oz	55
medium	1 oz	110
large	2½ oz	280
jumbo	4 oz	450
with nuts	1 oz	160
reduced fat	1 oz	140
coconut, chocolate covered	1 oz	160
fortune (Chinese)	1 cookie	30
fudge	1 oz	130
ginger snaps	4 cookies; approx 1 oz	120

*Average calories; calorie counts vary widely among brands and recipes. Cookie sizes also vary widely; for packaged cookies, read the label.

Food	Serving Size	Calories
Cookies *(continued)*		
graham crackers	5 pieces; 1 oz	150
low fat	4 pieces; approx 1 oz	110
chocolate covered	1 oz	120
hazelnut	4 pieces; 1 oz	150
lady fingers	1 piece	40
lemon	1 oz	110
macaroons	1 oz	110
marshmallow, chocolate covered	2 pieces; 1 oz	120
molasses	1 oz	120
newtons		
fig	2 pieces; 1 oz	110
fat free	2 pieces; 1 oz	90
other fruit	2 pieces; 1 oz	100
oatmeal, with raisins		
small	½ oz	50
medium	1 oz	95
large	2½ oz	240
fat free	1 oz	90
peanut butter	2 cookies; 1 oz	135
refrigerated cookie dough		
chocolate	1 oz	130

Food	Serving Size	Calories
Cookies (continued)		
refrigerated cookie dough (continued)		
chocolate chip	1 oz	140
oatmeal	1 oz	140
peanut butter	1 oz	120
sugar	1 oz	130
sandwich		
chocolate covered	1 cookie; approx ¾ oz	110
cream filled, chocolate	2 cookies; approx 1½ oz	160
double filled	2 cookies; 1 oz	140
reduced fat	3 cookies; approx 1 oz	130
cream filled, peanut butter	2 cookies; 1 oz	130
cream filled, vanilla	3 cookies; approx 1 oz	140
reduced fat	1 oz	130
shortbread	1 oz	140
shortcake	1 oz	120
sugar	1 oz	140
vanilla wafers	1 oz	150
reduced fat	1 oz	110
waffle	1 oz	160

Food	Serving Size	Calories

Frozen Desserts: Ice Cream, Ices, Yogurts, Sorbets*

Cones**

sugar	1 cone	50
waffle	1 cone	50

Ice Cream

banana nut	½ cup	170
butter pecan	½ cup	180
cherry vanilla	½ cup	130
chocolate	½ cup	170
low fat	½ cup	150
chocolate chip	½ cup	235
fudge	½ cup	280
bar, with chocolate coating	3½ oz bar	360
chocolate chip	½ cup	170
mint	½ cup	170
light	½ cup	140
cookie dough	½ cup	190

*Average calories; calorie counts vary widely among brands. Butterfat content of ice creams run from 0% (fat free), 4% (low fat), 6% (reduced fat) to 10% (regular) and 16%–20% for premium. This affects both calorie and fat counts. Read the label.

**Single scoops are generally 3 oz. Add ice cream portion to unfilled cone to obtain total calories.

Food	Serving Size	Calories
Frozen Desserts: Ice Cream, Ices, Yogurts, Sorbets _(continued)_		
coffee	½ cup	160
low fat	½ cup	116
macadamia nut brittle	½ cup	300
Neapolitan	½ cup	160
low fat	½ cup	110
peach	½ cup	130
low fat	½ cup	120
pecan praline	½ cup	200
peppermint	½ cup	150
pistachio	½ cup	170
rocky road	½ cup	180
rum raisin	½ cup	270
low fat	½ cup	130
sandwich	1	250
strawberry	½ cup	150
low fat	½ cup	110
vanilla	½ cup	160
low fat	½ cup	140
cookies and cream	½ cup	170
low fat	½ cup	145

Sweets and Desserts

Food	Serving Size	Calories

Frozen Desserts: Ice Cream, Ices, Yogurts, Sorbets
(continued)

vanilla *(continued)*

fudge	½ cup	160
fat free	½ cup	100
Swiss almond	½ cup	310
bar, with chocolate coating	3 ½ oz bar	330
bar, with chocolate and almond coating	3 ½ oz bar	320

Tofu-Based

berry	½ cup	190
"butter" pecan	½ cup	220
chocolate	½ cup	180
cookie crunch	½ cup	210
vanilla	½ cup	190
fudge	½ cup	190

Frozen Yogurt
hard, all flavors

low fat	½ cup	140
nonfat	½ cup	110

soft, all flavors

low fat	½ cup	120
nonfat	½ cup	100

Ices, Sherbets, and Sorbets

all flavors	½ cup	115

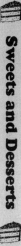

Sweets and Desserts

Food	Serving Size	Calories
Jams, Jellies, Preserves, and Spreads		
apple butter	I tbsp	35
fruit spread, all flavors	I tbsp	50
reduced calorie	I tbsp	20
jam, all flavors	I tbsp	50
jelly, most flavors	I tbsp	50
mint	I tbsp	60
strawberry	I tbsp	60
marmalade, all flavors	I tbsp	50
Pastries*		
apple brown Betty, home recipe	I cup	230
baklava	1⅓ oz	210
charlotte russe, home recipe	4 oz	325
cherry cobbler	4 oz	280
cinnamon bun	2 oz	230
reduced fat	2 oz	160
cream puff		
custard filled, home recipe	I puff; approx 4½ oz	335

*Average calories; calorie counts vary widely among brands and recipes.

Food	Serving Size	Calories
Pastries (continued)		
croissant		
plain, butter, small	1½ oz	180
large	2½ oz	300
almond	3½ oz	420
apple	3½ oz	250
chocolate	3½ oz	400
danish		
cheese	2½ oz	265
cinnamon	2½ oz	265
fruit	2½ oz	265
nut	2 oz	280
donut		
cake type	1	200
chocolate coated	1	205
sugared, glazed	1	195
jelly filled	1	215
holes	5 pieces; 2 oz	220
cruller, glazed	1	170
yeast type		
glazed	1	240
cream filled	1	305
jelly filled	1	290
éclair, custard filled, chocolate iced	3½ oz	240
strudel	2½ oz	195
sweet bun/roll (refrigerated)		
cheese	2 oz	235

Food	Serving Size	Calories
Pastries *(continued)*		
sweet bun/roll (refrigerated) *(continued)*		
cinnamon raisin	2 oz	225
cinnamon, iced	1½ oz	145
raisin nut	2 oz	195
toaster tarts		
apple cinnamon	1¾ oz	200
low fat	1¾ oz	190
blueberry	1¾ oz	200
low fat	1¾ oz	190
brown sugar cinnamon	1¾ oz	210
low fat	1¾ oz	190
cherry	1¾ oz	205
low fat	1¾ oz	190
chocolate	1¾ oz	200
low fat	1¾ oz	190
strawberry	1¾ oz	200
low fat	1¾ oz	190
turnovers		
apple	2 oz	170
blueberry	2 oz	165
cherry	2 oz	175
Pies and Pie Fillings*		
apple		
pie	⅛ 9" pie	410
filling	21 oz can	600

*Average calories; calorie counts vary widely among brands and recipes.
Pies are per serving; fillings are amount to fill an average pie.

Sweets and Desserts

Food	Serving Size	Calories
Pies and Pie Fillings (continued)		
banana cream	⅛ 9" pie	400
blackberry		
pie	⅛ 9" pie	360
filling	21 oz can	630
blueberry		
pie	⅛ 9" pie	360
filling	21 oz can	630
butterscotch		
pie	⅛ 9" pie	355
filling (see *Puddings and Gelatin*)		
cherry		
pie	⅛ 9" pie	485
filling	21 oz can	680
chocolate cream		
pie	⅛ 9" pie	400
filling (see *Puddings and Gelatin*)		
chocolate mousse	⅛ 9" pie	245
coconut cream		
pie	⅛ 9" pie	395
filling	20 oz can	700
coconut custard	⅙ 8" pie	270
egg custard	⅙ 8" pie	260

Sweets and Desserts

Food	Serving Size	Calories
Pies and Pie Fillings *(continued)*		
key lime	1/5 8" pie	380
lemon		
pie	1/4 8" pie	300
filling (see *Puddings and Gelatin*)		
meringue	1/6 9" pie	360
mincemeat		
pie	1/8 9" pie	475
filling	21 oz can	950
peach		
pie	1/8 9" pie	300
filling	21 oz can	600
pecan	1/8 9" pie	500
pineapple		
chiffon	1/8 9" pie	235
custard	1/8 9" pie	250
pumpkin		
pie	1/8 9" pie	315
filling	21 oz can	850
rhubarb	1/8 9" pie	300
strawberry		
pie	1/8 9" pie	185
strawberry rhubarb	1/6 8" pie	280
filling	21 oz can	630

Food	Serving Size	Calories

Pies and Pie Fillings (continued)

sweet potato	1/8 9" pie	245
vanilla cream pie	1/8 9" pie	350
filling (see *Puddings and Gelatin*)		

Pie Crusts and Shells*

plain

home recipe	9"	970
made from mix	9"	800
frozen	9"	650
graham cracker	9"	880
phyllo	1 sheet	55

puff

sheet	9 oz	1020
shell	1 shell; approx 1 1/2 oz	225

Puddings and Gelatin*

banana

made from mix

with whole milk	1/2 cup	155
with low fat milk	1/2 cup	145
ready to eat	5 oz	180
blancmange, home recipe	1/2 cup	140

*Average calories; calorie counts vary widely among brands and recipes.

Food	Serving Size	Calories
Puddings and Gelatin (continued)		
bread, home recipe	½ cup	210
butterscotch, ready to eat	4 oz	155
chocolate		
home recipe		
with whole milk	½ cup	220
with low fat milk	½ cup	205
made from mix		
with whole milk	½ cup	160
with low fat milk	½ cup	150
ready to eat	5 oz	190
fat free	4 oz	100
coconut cream		
made from mix		
with whole milk	½ cup	160
with low fat milk	½ cup	145
crème brûlée, home recipe	½ cup	400
crème caramel		
home recipe	½ cup	220
made from mix		
with whole milk	½ cup	150
with low fat milk	½ cup	135
custard		
baked, home recipe	½ cup	210

Sweets and Desserts

Food	Serving Size	Calories
Puddings and Gelatin (continued)		
custard (continued)		
made from mix		
with whole milk	½ cup	160
with low fat milk	½ cup	150
ready to eat	4 oz	155
flan		
home recipe	½ cup	220
made from mix		
with whole milk	½ cup	150
with low fat milk	½ cup	135
gelatin (made from mix)		
all flavors, regular	½ cup	85
all flavors, artificially sweetened	½ cup	10
lemon		
made from mix		
with whole milk	½ cup	170
with sugar, egg yolk, water	½ cup	165
ready to eat	5 oz	180
mousse, chocolate		
home recipe	½ cup	445
made from mix	½ cup	80
prune whip, home recipe	1 cup	205
rice		
home recipe	½ cup	215

Sweets and Desserts

Food	Serving Size	Calories

Puddings and Gelatin (*continued*)

rice (*continued*)
made from mix

with whole milk	½ cup	175
with low fat milk	½ cup	160
ready to eat	5 oz	230

tapioca

home recipe	½ cup	190

made from mix

with whole milk	½ cup	160
with low fat milk	½ cup	145
ready to eat	5 oz	170

vanilla

home recipe	½ cup	130

made from mix

with whole milk	½ cup	160
with low fat milk	½ cup	140
ready to eat	½ cup	145

Sauces and Toppings*

butterscotch	2 tbsp	130
caramel	2 tbsp	120
fat free	2 tbsp	100

chocolate

fudge	2 tbsp	145
hot fudge type	2 tbsp	130

*Average calories; calorie counts vary widely among brands and recipes.

Sweets and Desserts

Food	Serving Size	Calories

Sauces and Toppings *(continued)*

chocolate *(continued)*

mint, fat free	2 tbsp	110
syrup	2 tbsp	85
light	2 tbsp	50
topping	2 tbsp	110
marshmallow cream	2 tbsp	40
pineapple	2 tbsp	105
strawberry	2 tbsp	105
walnut syrup	2 tbsp	165

Sugars, Sweeteners, and Syrups

Note: All sugars, sweeteners, and syrups have 0 fat. They derive all of their calories from sugar, a carbohydrate.

corn syrup, dark, light, high fructose	1 tbsp	55
honey	1 tbsp	65
maple syrup	1 tbsp	52
molasses		
blackstrap	1 tbsp	45
dark or light	1 tbsp	60
pancake and waffle syrup	1 tbsp	55
light	1 tbsp	25

Sweets and Desserts

173

Food	Serving Size	Calories
Sugars, Sweeteners, and Syrups *(continued)*		
sorghum syrup	1 tbsp	60
sugar		
brown	1 cup packed	825
white	1 tsp	15
	1 tbsp	50
	1 cup	775
powdered (confectioners')	1 tbsp	30
	1 cup	120
sugar substitute	1 tsp	5

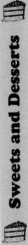

Food	Serving Size	Calories
Vegetables		
alfalfa sprouts	1 cup	10
artichoke		
whole	10 oz	150
hearts	1 oz	30
marinated	1 oz	20
Jerusalem (see *Jerusalem artichoke*)		
arugula	1/2 cup; approx 1/3 oz	5
asparagus		
fresh	6 spears; approx 3 oz	20
canned	1/2 cup	25
frozen	4 spears; approx 2 oz	15
avocado		
California	1	305
Florida	1	340
purée	1 cup	370
slices	1 cup	235
dip, guacamole (see *Snack Foods*)		
bamboo shoots, canned	1 cup	25
bean sprouts, mung, raw	1/2 cup; approx 2 oz	16
beets		
root		
whole, fresh, boiled	3 oz	35
canned	1/2 cup; approx 3 oz	25
pickled	1/2 cup; approx 4 oz	75

Food	Serving Size	Calories
Vegetables *(continued)*		
beets *(continued)*		
greens, boiled	½ cup	20
bell pepper (see *pepper*)		
bok choy		
raw	½ cup; approx 1 oz	5
cooked	½ cup; approx 3 oz	10
broccoli		
fresh, raw	1½ oz	12
fresh, boiled	2¾ oz	20
frozen, chopped, boiled	½ cup; approx 3¼ oz	25
Brussels sprouts, boiled	½ cup; approx 2¾ oz	30
cabbage		
Chinese, raw	½ cup, shredded	5
green		
raw	½ cup, shredded	9
boiled	½ cup, shredded	15
red		
raw	½ cup, shredded	9
boiled	½ cup, shredded	15
sweet and sour pickled	½ cup	100
Savoy (see *cabbage, green*)		
cole slaw	½ cup	40
capers	1 tbsp	5

Food	Serving Size	Calories
Vegetables *(continued)*		
carrot		
fresh, raw	1 medium; approx 2½ oz	30
boiled	½ cup, slices	25
canned	½ cup	15
frozen	½ cup	25
dried	1 oz	100
cassava, raw	3½ oz	120
cauliflower, fresh, frozen	½ cup, florets	15
celery	1 stalk	5
celery root (celeriac), raw	3½ oz	40
chard (see *Swiss chard*)		
chicory	½ cup; approx 3 oz	20
chives, chopped	1 oz	10
chiles (see *peppers*)		
collards, chopped, boiled	1 cup; approx 4½ oz	35
corn		
fresh		
on the cob	5½ oz, with cob	80
kernels	½ cup	90

Food	Serving Size	Calories
Vegetables *(continued)*		
corn *(continued)*		
canned		
in water	½ cup	65
cream style	½ cup	90
frozen	½ cup	65
hominy, canned	1 cup	115
cucumber	½ cup slices; approx 2 oz	10
eggplant, raw	½ cup	10
endive (chicory, whitloof)	½ cup	10
fennel, bulb, raw	1 cup, slices; approx 3 oz	25
garlic		
fresh, raw	1 clove	5
chopped, in oil	1 tsp	10
powder	1 tsp	10
ginger		
root, fresh	1 oz	20
root, pickled	1 oz	10
powder	1 tsp	6
green beans		
fresh, raw	½ cup	15
boiled	½ cup; approx 2 oz	20
canned	½ cup; approx 2 oz	14

Food	Serving Size	Calories
Vegetables *(continued)*		
green beans *(continued)*		
frozen	½ cup; approx 3 oz	25
green onions (see *scallions*)		
Jerusalem artichoke (sunchoke)	½ cup, slices	55
kale, chopped, boiled	½ cup	20
leek, chopped, raw	¼ cup; approx 1 oz	15
lentil sprouts, raw	½ cup	40
lettuce, all types	½ oz, shredded; 1 oz	5
lima beans		
fresh, boiled	½ cup	115
canned	½ cup	85
frozen	½ cup	85
dried (see *Beans*)		
mixed vegetables		
frozen	½ cup	55
canned	½ cup	40
mung bean, sprouts (see *bean sprouts*)		
mushrooms		
fresh, raw	½ cup; approx 1 oz	5
canned	½ cup; approx 3 oz	20
dried (shiitake)	1 oz	45

Food	Serving Size	Calories
Vegetables *(continued)*		
mustard greens, boiled	½ cup, chopped	10
okra		
raw	½ cup; approx 2 oz	15
boiled	½ cup; approx 3 oz	30
olives		
all types, small–large	1 olive	5
all types, jumbo–colossal	1 olive	10
oil cured	1 oz; approx 10 olives	70
onion		
fresh, raw		
whole	3 oz	10
chopped	½ cup	30
boiled	4 oz	12
small, frozen	½ cup; 4 oz	40
dried, flakes	¼ cup; ½ oz	45
fried rings, battered	2 oz	140
pickled, cocktail	1 tbsp	0
green (see *scallions*)		
palm, hearts	1 oz	10
parsley		
fresh	½ cup, chopped	11
dried	¼ tsp	0
freeze dried	1 tsp	1
root	1 oz	10

Vegetables and Dried Beans

Food	Serving Size	Calories
Vegetables (continued)		
parsnip		
raw	½ cup, slices	50
boiled	½ cup, slices	65
pea pods (see *snow peas*)		
peas, black-eye (see *Beans*)		
peas, green		
fresh, raw, shelled	½ cup	60
frozen	½ cup	60
canned, all types	½ cup	60
pepper		
hot, chile		
raw	1½ oz	20
green, canned	¼ cup	5
jalapeño, diced, canned	2 tbsp	5
sweet, green, red, yellow		
raw, whole	medium	20
raw, chopped	½ cup	15
frozen	1 cup	25
roasted	1 oz	10
roasted, in olive oil	1 oz	20
pimiento	1 tbsp	5
cherry, pickled	1 oz	10
plantain (see *Fruits*)		
pickles		
bread and butter	1 oz	20

Food	Serving Size	Calories
Vegetables (continued)		
pickles (continued)		
cornichons	1 oz	0
dill	1 oz	5
gherkins, sweet	1 oz	25
potato		
fresh, raw, without skin	4 oz	90
diced, peeled	1 cup	120
canned, without skin	½ cup	55
baked, microwaved, with skin	7 oz	220
boiled, with skin	4 oz	85
boiled, without skin	1 cup	135
au gratin	½ cup	160
fried, pan	3 oz	275
French-fried	2 oz	175
hash brown	½ cup	165
mashed		
home recipe, with milk and butter	½ cup	110
instant	½ cup	120
kugel	5 oz	300
pancake	1 oz	100
salad		
German style	½ cup	125
with mayo	½ cup	180
scalloped	½ cup	105
sweet (see *sweet potato*)		
pumpkin, canned, unsweetened	½ cup	40
pie mix (see *Sweets and Desserts: Pie Fillings*)		

Food	Serving Size	Calories
Vegetables *(continued)*		
radicchio	½ cup, shredded	5
radish	1 oz	5
rhubarb		
boiled, unsweetened	½ cup	35
boiled, sweetened	½ cup	140
rutabaga, boiled	½ cup, cubes	35
sauerkraut	½ cup	25
sweet and sour	½ cup	80
scallions	½ cup, chopped	15
shallot	1 tbsp, chopped	10
snow peas		
raw	3 oz	35
boiled	½ cup	35
frozen	3 oz	35
soybeans		
boiled	½ cup	130
sprouts	1 cup	100

soybean products
soy flour (see *Sweets and Desserts: Baking Ingredients*)
soy milk, tofu (see *Diet and Health Foods*)
soy sauce, miso (see *Extras*)
soynuts (see *Nuts and Seeds*)

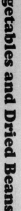

Vegetables and Dried Beans

Vegetables (continued)

spinach

fresh, raw	½ cup, chopped	5
canned, frozen	½ cup	25
creamed	½ cup	60

sprouts (see individual vegetable)

squash

summer: zucchini, yellow

raw	½ cup, sliced	15
boiled	½ cup	20

winter: acorn, butternut, hubbard

raw	½ cup, cubes	20
baked	½ cup, cubes	40
boiled, mashed	½ cup	40

string beans (see *green beans*)

sugar snap peas (see *snow peas*)

sunchoke (see *Jerusalem artichoke*)

sweet potato

raw	4 oz	135
baked, steamed	4 oz	115
mashed	1 cup	260
candied	3¾ oz	145
canned		
in light syrup	½ cup; 4 oz	120
in heavy syrup	½ cup; 4½ oz	125
chips (see *Snack Foods: Chips*)		

Vegetables and Dried Beans

Food	Serving Size	Calories
Vegetables *(continued)*		
Swiss chard, boiled	½ cup, chopped	20
tomatillo, raw	1 medium; approx 1 oz	10
tomato		
fresh, raw	1 medium; approx 4 oz	25
green	1 medium; approx 4 oz	30
boiled	½ cup	30
canned		
paste	2 tbsp	30
purée	1 cup	100
stewed	1 cup	80
whole, peeled	1 cup	50
sun dried	2 oz	140
in oil	1 cup	235
turnip		
raw	½ cup, cubed	20
boiled	½ cup	15
mashed	½ cup	20
water chestnuts, canned	½ cup	35
watercress	1 cup; 1 oz	5
yam (see *sweet potato*)		
zucchini (see *squash, summer*)		

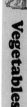
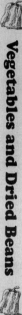

Food	Serving Size	Calories
Beans (dried, legumes)		
adzuki		
boiled	1 cup	295
canned, sweetened	1 cup	700
baked*	1 cup	380
black		
dried, uncooked	½ cup	315
boiled	½ cup	115
canned	½ cup	100
sauce (see *Extras: Sauces*)		
black-eye peas		
fresh, raw	½ cup	65
boiled	½ cup	80
dried	½ cup	195
boiled	½ cup	160
canned	½ cup	90
broad		
boiled	1 cup	185
canned	1 cup	180
chickpeas (garbanzo beans)		
dried, uncooked	¼ cup	170
boiled	1 cup	270
canned	1 cup	285
hummus (see *Snack Foods: Dips*)		

*Average calories; calorie count and serving size vary widely among brands.

Food	Serving Size	Calories

Beans (dried, legumes) *(continued)*

cow peas (see *black-eye peas*)

cranberry beans

dried, uncooked	½ cup	335
boiled	1 cup	240
canned	1 cup	215

garbanzo (see *chickpeas*)

great northern

dried, uncooked	½ cup	335
boiled	1 cup	210
canned	1 cup	300

kidney

dried, uncooked	½ cup	335
boiled	1 cup	225
canned	1 cup	210

lentils

dried, uncooked	½ cup	310
boiled	1 cup	230
sprouts (see *Vegetables*)		

lima

fresh (see *Vegetables*)		
dried, uncooked	½ cup	334
boiled	1 cup	210

Food	Serving Size	Calories

Beans (dried, legumes) *(continued)*

navy
dried, uncooked	½ cup	335
boiled	1 cup	260
canned	1 cup	300

peas, split
dried, uncooked	½ cup	115
boiled	1 cup	230

pinto
dried, uncooked	½ cup	335
boiled	1 cup	235
canned	1 cup	205

red
dried, uncooked	½ cup	335
boiled	1 cup	210
canned	1 cup	165

refried, canned	½ cup	150
fat free	½ cup	100

soy
dried, uncooked	1 cup	385
boiled	1 cup	300
roasted (see *Nuts and Seeds*)		
sauce (see *Extras: Condiments*)		
sprouts (see *Vegetables*)		
tofu (see *Health and Diet Foods*)		
tempeh (see *Health and Diet Foods*)		
miso (see *Extras: Flavorings*)		

Here is some space for you to add your own often-eaten foods and their calorie contents.

Food	Serving Size	Calories

Food	Serving Size	Calories

Food	Serving Size	Calories

Food	Serving Size	Calories